Endorsements

Pain is a worldwide problem that negatively affects individuals, families and society at large. Furthermore, we know that both work both paid and unpaid can convey significant benefits, but the ways that we work and the concept of work itself is rapidly changing. In this authoritative and superbly written book, Eccleston, Wainwright and colleagues explore the relationships between pain and work at multiple levels. The authors take a life-span approach to their subject providing an in-depth exploration of the effects of pain on occupation, where occupation is defined broadly as time spent in school, working at home, on the job and engaging in volunteer activities. The authors provide directions for future research and policy that, if enacted, could help to positively impact the lives of individuals living with pain, their family members and society. This book is essential reading for those interested in the problem of pain; the psychology of work; and occupational health.

Dr Cary Reid
Associate Professor of Medicine
Weill Cornell Medicine, New York, USA

Wainwright and Eccleston are to be congratulated on this comprehensive overview of pain in relation to education and work. The style is accessible and easy to read. Working with chronic pain now and in the future is brilliantly contextualised with a socio-historical account of work but the book also considers the implications of the changing world of work and the effect of the Gig economy. There are excellent insights into parenting, educating and employing individuals with pain that would be invaluable for anyone in those situations. Finally, this book channels the debate on "good work" and what this means for individuals and societies and highlights the importance of a workplace culture of "health and wellbeing" for the benefit of all of us, whether or not we have a long-term health condition.

Professor Karen Walker-Bone
Director of the National Centre of Excellence for
Musculoskeletal Health and Work, funded by
Versus Arthritis and the UK Medical Research Council

Work and pain
A lifespan development approach

Edited by

Elaine Wainwright
Senior Lecturer in Applied Psychology
Bath Spa University, and
Honorary Research Fellow
Centre for Pain Research
University of Bath, UK

Christopher Eccleston
Professor of Medical Psychology
Centre for Pain Research
The University of Bath, UK

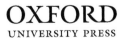
OXFORD
UNIVERSITY PRESS

OXFORD
UNIVERSITY PRESS

Great Clarendon Street, Oxford, OX2 6DP,
United Kingdom

Oxford University Press is a department of the University of Oxford.
It furthers the University's objective of excellence in research, scholarship,
and education by publishing worldwide. Oxford is a registered trade mark of
Oxford University Press in the UK and in certain other countries

Published in the United States of America by Oxford University Press
198 Madison Avenue, New York, NY 10016, United States of America

British Library Cataloguing in Publication Data

Data available

Library of Congress Control Number: 2019948416

ISBN 978–0–19–882827–3

Printed in Great Britain by
Ashford Colour Press Ltd, Gosport, Hampshire

Contents

Contributors

Stephen Bevan
Professor and Head of
HR Research Development,
Institute for Employment Studies, UK

Line Caes
Lecturer in Psychology,
Division of Psychology,
Faculty of Natural Sciences,
University of Stirling, UK

Michael Calnan
Professor of Medical Sociology,
School of Social Policy, Sociology,
and Social Research,
University of Kent, UK

Stephania Donayre Pimentel
Department of Psychology,
McGill University, Canada

Tom Douglass
ESRC Governing Scientific
Accountability RA and Doctoral
Researcher in Sociology,
School of Social Policy,
Sociology, and Social Research,
University of Kent, UK

Christopher Eccleston
Professor of Medical Psychology,
Centre for Pain Research,
The University of Bath, UK

Emma Fisher
Teaching Fellow,
Psychology Department,
The University of Bath, UK

Tiina Jaaniste
Head of Paediatric Pain and Palliative
Care Research Team, Department
of Pain and Palliative Care, Sydney
Children's Hospital, and dSchool
of Women's and Children's Health,
University of New South Wales,
Australia

Abbie Jordan
Senior Lecturer in Psychology,
Department of Psychology,
and Centre for Pain Research,
The University of Bath, UK

Deirdre Logan
Associate Professor of Psychology,
Department of Anesthesia,
Perioperative and Critical Care
Medicine, Children's Hospital Boston,
and Department of Psychiatry,
Harvard Medical School, USA

Chris J. Main
Professor of Clinical Psychology
(Pain Management),
Primary Care and Health Sciences,
Keele University, UK

Catherine Paré
Department of Psychology,
McGill University, Canada

William S. Shaw
Department of Family Medicine
and Community Health,
University of Massachusetts
Medical School, USA

Michael J. L. Sullivan
Professor of Psychology, Canada
Research Chair in Behavioural Health,
Department of Psychology, McGill
University, Canada

Jos Verbeek
Finnish Institute of Occupational Health,
Cochrane Work, Finland

Elaine Wainwright
Senior Lecturer in Applied Psychology,
Bath Spa University, and Honorary
Research Fellow, Centre for Pain
Research, University of Bath, UK

Section 1

Foundations

Chapter 1

Introduction

Elaine Wainwright and Christopher Eccleston

Introduction

Pain is one of the most significant health burdens of our time (Goldberg and McGee, 2011; Eccleston et al., 2018). Simultaneously, the ways we work are changing rapidly as we shape our working practices, and may feel shaped by them, alongside socio-political transformations. Debates about the nature of work in the West go back to at least Judeo-Christian narratives around the Garden of Eden—Adam and Eve are cast out of paradise, where they had been able to work in happiness, to beyond the garden gates, where they must till the lands in toil and pain.

As Grint (2005) discusses, work can be a symbol of personal value, and confer financial and social rewards, but it is also the punishment for original sin, and can include back-breaking labour camps or soul-destroying repetition. Work and pain are often bound together in the English language. 'Labour' can refer to work and childbirth, evoking images of effort and pain in both instances. 'Travail' also encapsulates ideas of work and pain in one word. It means 'painful or laborious effort' (Oxford Dictionaries Online, 2018). Its precise etymology is obscure but is known to stem from the mid-thirteenth century Old French word 'travail' meaning 'suffering; painful effort'. This in turn came from various vulgar and literary Latin routes including the Medieval Latin 'trepalium' meaning 'instrument of torture'. The duality inherent in 'labour' and 'travail' captures some of the fundamental issues of this book: is work good for people, including the many children and adults around the world who live with pain, or does it exacerbate or even cause painful problems? Can the same activity achieve respite from pain through engagement or produce more pain than would otherwise be suffered, depending on the many subjective and objective factors which make up the worker and their working environment?

The aim of this book is to provide an authoritative, thought-provoking analysis of the relationship between different forms of occupation (school, employment, later life production) and pain. We begin with a brief introduction to the aim of the text and what a consideration of work and pain can offer. We introduce our life-span approach and scope of the book, with its common structure, as each new chapter covers a particular element within our three core areas, Foundations, Investigations, and Interventions.

The effect that pain has on different occupations—schooling, home working, paid employment, voluntary occupations—throughout the life span, is critical to how people live and the goals and value of the lives they live. This is a particularly important time to reinvigorate engagement in this field. First, there is now a growing understanding that pain is a major part of childhood, and for many people a defining feature. The direct effects of pain on academic and social development, and the indirect effects on parents in both the labour of parenting and the ability of parents to undertake paid labour, make this a valuable topic for discussion. Second, the global changes in the content and delivery of work, the economic and technical changes of what we consider to be work, including—for the West—the rise of emotional labour whereby workers regulate their own and others' emotions, and insecure 'gig' working, have not been considered from a pain perspective. And finally, the radically changing age demographic in the twenty-first century with larger populations of people living and working into later life, undertaken often in the context of one or more painful long term conditions, requires a new consideration of later life working. These are just three examples of why we believe there is a need for a modern psychosocial consideration of pain and labour.

We take a life-span approach, exploring what it means to be working, from childhood to old age, within the context of pain. We consider work in its broadest sense of being occupied, at school, work, home, and in later life production. We elucidate how occupation interacts with suffering, and the reduction or exacerbation of that suffering, for people in pain. The book is designed to appeal to anyone interested in: pain in itself; suffering due to pain and ameliorating that suffering; the psychology of work; occupational health, and how policy intersects with systems and people's lived experience in the context of work and pain.

The goals of this text are:

1. To introduce a life-span approach to interactions between living with pain and being 'occupied'
2. To explore the ambivalence inherent in work which can be both rewarding and punishing, and how this may intersect with the pain experience
3. To discuss existing data on children and adults in pain in conjunction with their 'work' and to consider what we do not yet know
4. To analyse the policy context around return to work via our life-span perspective
5. To argue for a transdisciplinary approach to the study of pain and work over the life span

Each chapter covers a particular element within our three core areas: Foundations, Investigations and Interventions. We now briefly describe the aims and scope of these sections.

Section 1: Foundations

The two chapters in the 'Foundations' section consider first what is work, and second what is pain, per se, and then in relation to occupation. In Chapter 2, Michael Calnan and Tom Douglass critically consider what constitutes work in the twenty-first century. They chart a brief history and sociology of occupation, arguing that whilst changes in the form, experience, and understanding of work might in some ways be significant, they are more piecemeal than may first appear. They present a nuanced discussion of the contemporary face of employment in the twenty-first century, exploring and debating the gig economy, the impacts of complex technologies and automation, home working, and longer working lives. Finally, Calnan and Douglass discuss the implications and consequences of (the partial) changes in the nature and form of work for disease, illness, and health. In Chapter 3, Elaine Wainwright reviews the nature of pain, discussing when does pain occur and for how long, how is it thought about, how can we and should we think about it, and how does it relate to work? This includes a description of the epidemiology with a focus on interference caused by pain, and the evidence for the impact of pain across the life span.

Section 2: Investigations

This section analyses what we know regarding learning about pain, expectations of pain management, and setting the course for pain. In Chapter 4, Abbie Jordan and Tiina Jaaniste consider family labour, focusing on the impact of child pain on parental mental health and parenting behaviour, the intergenerational transmission of pain behaviour and pain learning, and the impact of parental pain on the parenting role. In Chapter 5, Line Caes and Deirdre Logan consider the importance of schooling for learning but also for social and emotional development. They discuss how chronic pain, and associated psychosocial factors, go beyond school absenteeism and also influence school engagement, executive functioning skills crucial for academic performance, and social skills development. They consider how teachers and organizations might help young people, and propose a new 'bio-psycho-social' model of school functioning in young people with chronic pain.

In Chapter 6, Emma Fisher and Christopher Eccleston consider emerging adulthood. The emergence of the millennial generations and their different relationships with work and working have been explored in occupational psychology but not in health psychology. Fisher and Eccleston consider what it means to have chronic pain as a millennial. They explore what we know from the research on the millennial generation and the world in which they exist, briefly touching on the sociological, economic, and technological context of this generation. They then discuss the expectations and values of millennials at work before focusing on millennials and health. Fisher and Eccleston examine how health has changed over the generations, how millennials access health care, and then focus on chronic pain. They end by discussing the difficult transition from paediatric to adult services, and by providing future directions in this field.

In Chapter 7, Jos Verbeek considers workers with occupational pain and the occupational pain workforce. The traditional world of work is explored, in particular how the changing patterns of work outlined in Chapter 2, such as the rise of mechanization, of emotional labour, and changing expectations of work, affect first how people and organizations respond to pain in the workforce, and second how the workforce of pain management specialists is responding. Occupational pain is defined as pain that is caused by occupational activities. This additional diagnosis of occupational origin is important for pain management, prevention, and compensation. Finally, in the Investigations section, Christopher Eccleston in Chapter 8 critically considers the role of later life in interactions between pain and work. Given that people are living for longer, the amount of time out of traditional occupational workforces in later life is growing. Multimorbidity and pain are a feature of later and end of life, but how this affects occupation (however rewarded or remunerated) has not been explored. The wisdom of older age is a major source of knowledge and practice, and this will re-viewed as source of evidence for the development of this new phase of knowledge and later life working in the context of pain.

Section 3: Interventions

In this section, we critically review what individuals can change, what workplaces can do and how governments can innovate to try to maximize workability for pain sufferers in the context of current working practices. In Chapter 9, Michael Sullivan, Stephanie Pimentel, and Catherine Paré examine the considerable research that has been conducted on trajectories of recovery. There is great interest in this area, not least because individuals who remain work-disabled at 3-months post-injury have a high likelihood of permanent disability. The failure to identify reliable medical or physical predictors of prolonged work disability has prompted consideration of non-medical variables that might be influencing return-to-work outcomes following musculoskel-etal injury. Sullivan, Pimentel, and Paré discuss what is currently known about psy-chological risk factors for problematic recovery following musculoskeletal injury. They consider cognitive variables such as self-efficacy and pain catastrophizing, mental health variables such as depression, and the implications of such variables on how we design and execute interventions. They also consider what we do not yet know in this area and provide some much-needed future research directions.

In Chapter 10, Chris Main and William Shaw consider the role of the employer in re-sponding to pain-related work limitations, and the challenges of implementing change in an occupational environment often focused sharply on profit and the avoidance of litigation. Main and Shaw begin with a description and attempted quantification of the burden of pain-related work limitations. They then offer a review of the major or-ganizational processes, the influence of management structures and prognostic factors before considering workplace interventions, and the influence of health/social policy. They conclude with a series of recommendations for an integrated approach to the management of PWL. In Chapter 11, Stephan Bevan considers when policy works and when does it not. The focus is on pain across occupied life and the success or otherwise of policy attempts to be relevant to people in the context of changing working lives. What different approaches can we take? The analysis here concerns governmental and political attempts to legislate, innovate, and motivate both the workforce and em-ployers to alter working practices to promote employability, workplace health, and productivity.

Finally, in the Discussion chapter, Elaine Wainwright and Christopher Eccleston summarize and review the findings from across all contributing chapters, and discuss the emergent themes. We know that the need to manage pain is unlikely to reduce dramatically in the near future. There is of course uncertainty regarding what new technologies and interventions we might develop, and how these might map onto the individual child enrolled in school, or millennial emerging into adulthood, or patient going to see the doctor, or employee trying to sustain their working life. However, we bring together the findings of this book to develop a conceptual and analytical map of the forces of change in work, occupation, and pain management. We suggest future directions for research and policy which could positively impact on our lives.

References

Eccleston, C., Wells, C., and Morlion, B. (eds) (2018) *European Pain Management.* Oxford: OUP.

Goldberg, D., and McGee, S. (2011) Pain as a global health priority. *BMC Public Health,* **11**, 770.

Grint, K. (2005) *The Sociology of Work: an Introduction.* 3rd edn. Bristol: Polity Press.

Oxford Dictionaries. (2018) Online. Available at: https://www.oed.com/search?searchType=dictionary&q=travail&_searchBtn=Search [Accessed 2 August 2019].

Chapter 2

A socio-historical account of work: Change, continuity, and the consequences

Michael Calnan and Tom Douglass

Introduction

What is work? Who does it and what does it mean to these people? What forms might work take and has the nature of work changed? Focusing particularly on the British context, from a sociological perspective this chapter will establish what work looks like in the twenty-first century and if/how this might be different from the past. In engaging with these key sociological questions, this chapter traces a social history of work and espouses the overarching argument that changes in the form, experience, and understanding of work, whilst certainly significant and pronounced in some ways, are, overall, partial and piecemeal. The chapter begins with a brief look at the consequences of industrialization and the organization of work in pre-industrial and industrial societies. It then moves to a detailed consideration of developments from the 1970s onwards, exploring, first, the end of the 'golden age' of work and core factors shaping the face of work in the final decades of the twentieth century (though emphasizing both continuity and change). The chapter then discusses the contemporary face of employment in the twenty-first century, exploring and debating the gig economy, the impacts of complex technologies and automation, home working, and longer working lives. Finally, the implications and consequences of (the partial) changes in the nature and form of work for disease, illness, and health are discussed.

The consequences of industrialization

As Volti (2012, pp. 39–54) overviews, for thousands of years humans were able to survive and sustain themselves nomadically through hunting and gathering, and then eventually through more geographically fixed agricultural and artisanal techniques. In the eighteenth century, though slow and distributed in its unfolding, the industrial revolution brought about significant social and economic change. There were major technological advances (e.g. the emergence and utilization particularly of machinery, such as looms, and new power sources, such as steam) and changes in the organization and form of work and labour. New power sources and machines were located in new production environments, the factory or mill (rather than the fields or the home) where large numbers of workers could be housed in one physical space. Indeed, 'by the second half of the nineteenth century, the industrial landscape was dotted with textile mills, meatpacking plants, steel mills, shoe factories, and other productive enterprises that put large numbers of workers under one roof' (Volti, 2012, p. 40). Such spaces certainly reflected new technological requirements but also the necessity of organizing and supervising large numbers of workers tolerating poor working conditions and with no personal stake in the efficiency or effectiveness of the factory's production processes other than their need to earn at least a subsistence wage. Work at this time was highly physically demanding, monotonous, long, subject to strict rules, and often extremely dangerous. In contrast to the organization of hunter-gather societies (with limited social stratification) and agricultural societies (with land as the source of power and wealth), developing capitalist economic relationships and arrangements (where ownership of productive means became the source of wealth and power) underpinned work at this time and were facilitated by vast and quickly occurring urbanization. As time progressed, the assembly line in the later stages of the nineteenth century and the early parts of the twentieth century was perhaps the most significant development. Most famously associated with American industrialist and automobile manufacturer Henry Ford, the assembly line, with workers conducting a specific task over and over, was designed to cut productions costs to make automobiles (and other manufactured products) affordable for the masses, to cut production time, and to make manufacturing more efficient.

The end of the 'golden age' and post-industrialization?

Fast forward to the decades following the Second World War and the continuing growth and development of industrial society in the aftermath of war had resulted in the dawn of a 'golden age' of seemingly limitless affluence and economic growth, full employment, workers' rights, and high levels of social security (Strangleman and Warren, 2007, pp. 126–7; Wainwright and Calnan, 2002, p. 125). This employment 'golden age' emerging from the post-war consensus was rooted in Keynesian economics, with its emphasis on state planning and increased investment through public expenditure, and lasted until the downturn of the mid-1970s—with the power of trade unions and workers and their pursuits of ever more 'generous' employment conditions blamed for economic collapse (at least in commentary from those on the right of the political spectrum). This economic downturn alongside the election of a Conservative government led by Margaret Thatcher in 1979 ended the era of social democracy and ushered in the New Right and neoliberalism—throwing off constraints to the operation of free markets. As Wainwright and Calnan (2002, pp. 124–7) discuss, Mrs Thatcher's government can be argued to have quickly and dramatically altered employment conditions in Britain in a number of ways, seemingly favouring the interests of employers over workers. Certainly 'inefficient' traditional industries revolving around manufacturing or extraction went into decline or were closed with vastly significant impacts on communities centred around steel, coal mining, or shipbuilding. Indeed, as a result of the process of deindustrialization more than 4 million jobs in manufacturing were lost between 1971 and 1995 (from 7,890,000 to 3,845,000) (Noon and Blyton 2002, p. 34). Equally, removed (for some) were traditional expectations of a job for life and gone, at least partially, was Fordist imagery of assembly line routine and predictability. Alongside high levels of unemployment for former industrial workers, movement in Britain at this time towards a post-industrial society meant shifts in employment towards service jobs and jobs utilizing information technologies. Deindustrialization and the creation of jobs in the service sector were also strongly gendered—with the decline of manufacturing and extraction industries signalling unemployment primarily for men and the growth of new low status and low pay jobs for women (Strangleman and Warren, 2007, pp. 136–7). Finally, in the interests of making Britain competitive in the global market, increasingly workers also needed to be flexible and multiskilled, to perform an array of tasks, to accept zero-hour and short-term contracts, and to retrain and/or relocate as dictated by the needs of the market. Workers were also subjected to new managerial approaches facilitated by information technology aiming to boost productivity and to control quality.

Some sociological narratives have emphasized vast changes in the availability and form of work as well as meaning and identity found in work as Western society appears to move beyond modernity and industrial forms of capitalism. As Strangleman (2007, pp. 83–8) reviews, core themes in sociological accounts are of the vast pace of change, of the quantitatively and qualitatively different nature of work and what is desired and required from work, and of loss (loss of stability and predictability, loss of a job for life, the loss of a specific society and specific modes of belonging) (see Gorz, 1999; Sennett, 1998). Other themes are of work in the past as the central aspect of life and where meaning was found, but that increasingly identity is derived from and meaning found in what one consumes (Bauman, 1998). Additionally, work is thematized as uncertain and insecure, reflecting but also furthering the risk society (Beck, 2000). And further, we find narratives of individualization, with work in the past considered collective but becoming increasingly individualized, and of fragmentation, with the traditional conception of a career replaced by a portfolio of jobs and pieces of work (Bauman, 1998; Beck, 2000; see also Strangleman, 2007, p. 88).

As these discussions indicate, there have certainly been strong narratives from prominent social theorists (though also at political and public levels) about changes in the form and experience of work. However, another narrative suggests that change is perhaps better conceived of as partial and piecemeal with certain aspects of change more pronounced than others, and that an 'all change' approach lacks nuance. Strangleman (2007, p. 100) argues that notions such as no job can last forever, all employment security has been lost, or that no real meaning can be found in work anymore, are overstated claims. Certainly, deindustrialization is an important process, but it also creates a sense that no industrial work remains. For example, in 2007 the UK still had 3.5 million permanent and temporary jobs in manufacturing (Inman, 2018). Caution is also needed when lamenting relatively uncritically or engaging in a sort of 'smokestack nostalgia' (Cowie and Heathcott, 2003), about the decline of industrial work, much of which was dirty, hard, and damaging (Strangleman and Warren, 2007, p. 135). Furthermore, the 1945–1970s period was a relatively unusual stage of growth, stability, and security in the longer history of work (Strangleman, 2007, p. 95). Wainwright and Calnan (2002, pp. 127–36) also show how the average length of the working week actually fell from the mid-1970s from 39.2 down to 35.5 hours as the century closed. On one level, this confuses and complicates discussions of change as detrimental to the interests of workers. However, such figures themselves conceal a more nuanced picture, with, for example, average paid and unpaid overtime increasing slightly in the 1990s, though with important occupational differences reflecting diminished employment in blue collar and non-professional and non-managerial jobs. Similarly, job tenure at the end of the twentieth century had only diminished slightly compared with decades earlier in the century, but, importantly, seemingly impacted the young more than the old (Wainwright and Calnan, 2002). Moreover, intensification in work did seem to have risen by the end of the twentieth century when considering changes in work effort reflecting effort demanded by the job and the source of work pressure (Green, 2001); however, separating perceptions of intensification from cultural aspects, such as moral ideals around work ethic or concerns about work–life balance, that have shifted over time, is potentially difficult to achieve methodologically. Finally, though multiskilling, flexibility, dynamic forms of team working, and even home working might have held opportunity to empower workers and enhanced the experience of work as compared to the monotony of the production line, capitalist logics (though reconstituted and sped up) still underpin work, workers continue to sell their labour, and control over work processes and outputs remains largely beyond workers (Wainwright and Calnan, 2002).

Work patterns in the twenty-first century

More recent changes in working and employment patterns in the twenty-first century are suggestive of further change (though there are also aspects of continuity and/or hyperbolic arguments about change that are difficult to assess). For example, the manufacturing sector in Britain has further shrunk by 600,000 jobs (Inman, 2018). There also appears to be increasing precariousness of work (at least for some groups). For example, this is illustrated by the growth of the so-called gig economy (Lexis Nexus, 2015), which is a label to encompass the idea of short-term, unpredictable, informal working arrangements exemplified by delivery workers or Uber drivers.[1] Nearly 3 million people in the UK work in the gig economy (Department for Business, Energy and Industrial Strategy, 2018).

Other developments relate to the implications of the increasing use of complex technologies at work such as in the application of artificial intelligence and the use of robots, which is perhaps beginning to transform the nature of relations between workers and technology. For example, Ford (2015, p. 10) suggests that developments in this area may 'ultimately challenge one of our most basic assumptions about technology: that *machines are tools* that increase the productivity of workers. Instead, machines themselves are turning into workers, and the line between the capability of

---

[1] The 'gig economy' is not necessarily a novel term because musicians and other creative professionals have for some time described their work in the same way—although its spread into various industries, even white collar institutions such as universities, is more distinctive and indicative of change.

labour and capital is blurring as never before' [emphasis in the original]. According to Ford (2015), this will not just affect low skilled occupations but also those with relatively high skills and non-routine occupations will become routine work. It is claimed this development will lead to a further widening of social inequalities by reinforcing the enhancement of the position of the financial elite with their control over resources. However, the extent to which such developments have been and will be significant in terms of changing work patterns is difficult to assess, particularly given the current level of hyperbole about its potential impact.

However, there are more obvious consequences of developments in new technology (amongst many, the laptop, the smart phone, real time team collaboration tools, and social media), further exacerbating trends with a longer history, such as increasing homeworking, working away from an office and self-employment. There is evidence of an increasing shift towards homeworking not just amongst the self-employed but also amongst employees. For example, in 2002, no less than one in ten workers either worked mainly at home or used their home as a base. In addition, the Labour Force Survey shows that a further 1.2 million workers spent a shorter period of time—one full day of their working week—carrying out paid work at home. This comprised 4% of the working population in the UK in 2002, representing an increase of one-sixth over the 1997 equivalent figure. Overall these data suggest that in 2002 one in every eight (13%) of workers in the UK used their home to some extent as their place of work each week (around 3.8 million people) (Felstead et al., 2005). This trend has continued and by the mid-2010s, home working had risen to more than 4 million people, with more than 60% of these people self-employed (BBC, 2014).

Younger people in particular currently appear to be moving more into a precarious working environment (Standing, 2011) as the relationship between education and work also appears to have changed structurally. For example, the orthodox view tends to characterize the youth labour market in terms of a hierarchy of sectors which relate to education's institutional structure, for example, attendance at universities leading on to graduate jobs and attendance at colleges of further education leading to skilled work through apprenticeships, and the lack of either higher or further education being associated with semi or unskilled work (Brown et al., 2011). Theories of human capital (the performance of people and their potential in the organization) might thus predict that the more educated workers will be more productive and hence their incomes will be higher (Brown et al., 2011). Yet in the UK, as a recent Office of National Statistics report highlights, underemployment amongst graduates rose from 37% in 2001 to 47% in June 2013. In 2017, about half of recent graduates were in non-graduate occupations (ONS, 2017). Thus, the basic assumptions of the knowledge economy that the more younger people are skilled, the more likely they are to get highly skilled jobs has not proved to be a valid one despite younger people being more qualified than ever before (Mann and Huddleston, 2017). One explanation for this trend highlights the impact of globalization and the associated marketization, deregulation and inequality which tend to go with it. There is an apparent mismatch between expectations and employment, according to Brown et al. (2011) who argue that there is a global auction for highly skilled jobs in which those who are cheapest often win. The authors show that the competition for highly skilled jobs is now a worldwide competition—an auction for cut-priced brainpower—fuelled by an explosion of higher education across the world and a significant shift in power privileging corporate bosses and emerging economies. There are processes of standardizing, digitizing, and exporting what was once high-skilled knowledge work—what the authors call *digital Taylorism,* which is a modern version of scientific management. These structural changes in the operation of the youth labour market, as Mann and Huddleston (2017) suggest, have implications for education and training, and there are three key elements. First, the increasing complexity of the labour market has required greater levels of more authentic careers provision. Second, increasing competition where school to work transitions have become more fragmented with young people expecting that they leave education with higher levels of skills and with resilience to compete for employment opportunities. Finally workplace change where an increasing number of jobs demand not just knowledge itself, but also its effective application in new situations, drawing on skills often delivered by schools as enterprise education (Mann and Huddleston, 2017).

At the other end of the spectrum (and importantly in terms of the life course approach advocated by this book), working lives in the twenty-first century also seem to be expanding. In 2008 the average retirement age for men was 64.6 years old—the oldest age since 1984 (Vickerstaff, 2010, p. 873). Many people, particularly amongst the highly educated, those with high status jobs, and those with high salaries, also appear to be strongly attached to their jobs and even when retiring retain an interest in continuing paid or unpaid work (McNair, 2006). The average retirement age is likely to only further increase in the coming decades as State Pension age rises (to 66 by 2020 and to 67 in the late 2020s).

The discussion so far has focused primarily on paid work, but what of unpaid work—or work that takes the form of household labour, maintenance and repair, transport, shopping, and adult and child care, or various forms of voluntary work? Women in particular are involved in a combination of paid and unpaid work and retain the majority of the domestic burden. For example, recent evidence from the Office of National Statistics (2016) suggests that in 2015 women carried out, on average, 60% more unpaid work than men. On average, men do 16 hours of unpaid work a week, compared to 26 hours for women.

Work, the body, and health

A sociological analysis of the continuities and changes in patterns of work and employment has been offered in previous sections of this chapter. In this final part, the implications and consequences of the (partial) changes to the form and availability of work since the 1980s for illness and health will briefly be discussed as a way to begin and contextualize discussions held in the rest of this book.

Those concerned with occupational health (Wilde, 2016) suggest that the combination of precarity, low pay, compromised rights, bad work, and a lack of access to meaningful occupational health support means that those employed in the gig economy are vulnerable to an elevated risk of ill health, particularly a risk of poor mental health. Precarious work, it is suggested, will cause people to fall ill (Mireia et al., 2017) and then potentially into long-term sickness absence and disability, with the associated costs to health-care provision, damaged families, and weakened communities (Wilde, 2016). Pilgrim (2014) supports this assertion and points out that studies looking at the relationship between work and mental health suggest that the worst mental health scores are not found in the unemployed but in those in insecure employment, for example, low wages, poor task control, and poor job security. This position is elaborated on by Wilde (2016) who links the social epidemiological models of work stress, that is an interaction between degree of control, extent of demand, and level of support to the position of the gig worker: 'The work is low control as there is no certainty of work from one 'gig' to the next... The work is low support because working relationships are not consistent. The work is also high demand as they regularly pay under the minimum wage so requiring people to work too many hours merely to get by and feed their families' (Wilde, 2016, p. 1).

Deindustrialization and the decline of the manufacturing industry and manual work in high-income countries like the UK have meant that patterns of work-related disease and injury have changed. Hence, those diseases associated with industrialization such as accidents, injuries, and work-related illnesses, including those physical health problems associated with occupational hazards, pollutants, and carcinogens, although still prevalent, appear to be in decline. In contrast, it has been argued that there has been the development of a new wave of work-related illness. These include 'illnesses', sometimes referred to as contested illnesses (Dumit, 2006), for instance stress, musculoskeletal disorders, such as low back pain or upper limb pain (e.g. repetitive strain injury), and diffuse non-specific fatigue syndromes such as fibromyalgia or chronic fatigue syndrome. This has led some authors (Baxter et al., 2010) to make a conceptual distinction between illness and disease in occupational disorders where illness is a subjective state and disease is a pathological process that at least in theory might be open to objective external verification. The former types of condition do not seem to fit neatly into the exposure–response epidemiological paradigm which has been traditionally associated with the identification of the risk of occupational hazards and their prevention or management. The difficult but fundamental question is about understanding the relationship between the social and the biological and identifying the pathways or mechanisms which might link them. The basic question is how workers' interpretations and experiences become embodied or as Wainwright and Calnan (2002) state 'become written on the body' and sometimes manifest themselves both in mental and physical health problems.

It might be assumed that this new wave of work-related illnesses, such as work stress, is directly determined by the deterioration of working conditions, for example, increasing job insecurity. However, such an assumption has been contested by some authors (Wainwright and Calnan, 2002) who explore the question of whether the claims of the transformation of work during the 1980s, which were particularly argued to have involved a shift away from the interests of workers, also led to damage to workers' health. As noted earlier, they suggest that the narrative of the deterioration of working conditions might have been over exaggerated and point to evidence that average job tenure had changed little but that the redistribution of insecurity towards the middle classes led to a higher media profile for this 'problem'. Similarly, they argue that the proposition that there was an increase has occurred in the length of the working week is not necessarily evidence based. In relation to work intensification, they argue that the evidence of rising work effort from the mid-1980s might be equally the product of the dominant culture along with objective working conditions, given that most of the data are based on self-report, which might reflect the existence of a culture that privileges the moral ideal of the highly motivated, flexible, high-performing worker. In terms of the rise of managerialism and control, Wainwright and Calnan (2002) also argue that the more significant change is the extent to which managers have attempted to instil corporate values and have embedded their managerial worldview into the minds of their employees. The aim is to increase self-governance and self-surveillance, increase productivity, and undermine collective oppositional activities such as trade unionism.

This leads to the overall thesis of these authors that the so-called epidemic of work stress might be said to be more a reflection of a cultural shift. The collapse of the trade union movement, according to these authors, means that there are limited collective solutions available, leading to the individualization and subsequent medicalization of workers' problems. It must be emphasized here that the position of the occupational health service at the interface between industry and the health service and the conflicting pressures of the economic imperative of a profit motive and altruistic concerns with workers' health significantly shaped its development. Sociological theories of medical professionalism (Calnan, 2015) suggest that the key to the enhancement and maintenance of professional status, power, and authority is being able to secure and maintain a large degree of professional autonomy and discretion. Such a position is difficult to obtain in this particular organizational context and clinical setting so as a branch of medicine, it appears to be low status, along with other branches associated with public and environmental health (Ross, 2012), at least compared to those specialisms more firmly based in the clinical setting of the hospital. However, Wainwright and Calnan (2002) argue that state regulatory agencies such as the Health and Safety Executive (HSE) and legislation such as Health and Safety at Work provide a bridge between the concerns of the individual worker and the collective interests of the workforce as a whole, as for traditional problems at work to become legitimate, health and safety issues at work must be transformed into the causes of physical or mental harm to the worker. The concept of stress has been seen as fundamental to this transformation. The medicalized discourse of work stress has enabled the management of individual worker's problems when no collective solution has been available.

This approach has led to some focus on what workers do about their problems (Dodier, 1994) and the social meaning of sickness absence. One of the common criticisms of the medicalization thesis is that it is over deterministic. However, there is research evidence of resistance to medical labels, particularly in the context of mental health due to the fear and shame of being weak and inadequate (Wainwright and Calnan, 2002). However, other authors argue the contrary and portray sickness absence (Lipsedge and Calnan, 2010) as a form of resistance in terms of a covert form of acting out of indignation and anger and that workers have 'good' and serious reasons for entering the sick role. It reflects the notion that medicalization should be seen as neutral concept having both gains and losses. Employees may use their diagnostic label as a strategy for combating their feelings of being undervalued or exploited. It creates an identity for these employees. This is not an easy option to take, however, as the authors point out, given the moral imperative to be resilient and to continue to work.

The above authors have also suggested that there is another more recent discourse which highlights the more positive aspects of work and employment which is the discourse on well-being (Wainwright and Calnan, 2012). The basic premise is that being employed is good for people's heath. Work, according to some sociologists (Strangleman, 2007), still provides structure and meaning in people's lives despite uncertainty/insecurity. However, evidence from the negative experience of unemployment suggests that that there have been winners and losers in terms of the consequences of contemporary working patterns and conditions. For example, McIvor (2013) argues that recently there has been a polarization of experience and working lives are being divided into a privileged group with high earnings and rewarding jobs and a marginalized, low paid, and insecure segment. Inequalities have persisted and been recast around work enrichment and work deprivation.

Wainwright and Calnan (2012) suggest that the rise of the well-being discourse is increasingly favoured as a way of understanding the relationship between work and health. Certainly, the notion of well-being is a nebulous one and its conceptualization has been informed by a number of different disciplines. However, Wainwright and Calnan (2012) suggest that it might be a more useful sociological concept than the work stress phenomenon and propose that it should be theoretically grounded in the social determinants of illness action and resilience. This sociological narrative of work stress emphasizes the social-cultural construction of the phenomenon. It has some explanatory power but there is an alternative realist narrative (Sennett, 2006; Standing 2011) which also might have some resonance in terms of explaining the impact and consequences of more recent changes in work patterns. The precarious nature of some work clearly has implications for financial security and there is strong evidence of a link between material deprivation, both absolute and relative, and poorer health outcomes. Both unemployment and poor employment are threats to mental health, implying certain types of employment and work might be positive for mental health.

Conclusion

This chapter has provided a socio-historical account of patterns of working in Britain. It has considered the extent to which there has been continuity or significant changes in forms of working and the nature of work and it has considered the impact of recent developments such as the emergence of the gig economy and new technologies, such as those associated with artificial intelligence and increased automation. The overall argument suggests that while some aspects of change are significant the overall picture of work in the twenty-first century reflects partial and piecemeal change. However, though resisting an 'all change' perspective, as the final section of this chapter has indicated, work in the twenty-first century has unique consequences for both the understanding and experience of health and illness.

References

Baxter, P., Aw, T., Cockcroft, A., Durrington, P., and Harrington, J. (2010) The changing face of occupational disease. In: Baxter, P., Aw, T., Cockcroft, A., Durrington, P., and Harrington, J. (eds) *Hunter's Diseases of Occupation*. 10th edn. London: Hodder Arnold, 24–9.

Bauman, Z. (1998) *Work, Consumerism and the New Poor*. Buckingham: Open University Press.

BBC News (2014) ONS: Record numbers working from home. Online. Available at: https://www.bbc.co.uk/news/business-27694938

Beck, U. (2000) *The Brave New World of Work*. Cambridge: Polity.

Brown, P., Lauder, H., and Ashton, D. (2011) *The Global Auction: The Broken Promises of Education, Jobs and Incomes*. Oxford: Oxford University Press.

Calnan, M. (2015) Eliot Freidson: Sociological narratives of professionalism and modern medicine. In: Collyer, F. (ed.) *The Palgrave Handbook of Social Theory in Health, Illness and Medicine*. Basingstoke: Palgrave Macmillan, 287–305.

Cowie, J., and Heathcott, J. (eds) (2003) *Beyond the Ruins: The Meaning of Deindustrialization*. New York: Cornell University Press.

Department for Business, Energy and Industrial Strategy. (2018) The characteristics of those in the gig economy. Final report. Online. Available at: https://assets.publishing.service.gov.uk/government/uploads/system/uploads/attachment_data/file/687553/The_characteristics_of_those_in_the_gig_economy.pdf

Dodier, N. (1994) Expert medical decisions in occupational medicine: A sociological analysis of medical judgement. *Sociology of Health and Illness*, **16**, 489–574.

Dumit, J. (2006) Illnesses you have to fight to get: Facts as forces in uncertain emerging illnesses. *Social Science and Medicine*, **62**, 577–90.

Felstead, A., Jewson, N., and Walters, S. (2005) The shifting locations of work: New statistical evidence on the spaces and places of employment. *Work, Employment and Society*, **19**, 415–31.

Ford, A. (2015) *Rise of the Robots: Technology and the Threat of a Jobless Future*. New York: Basic Books.

Inman, P. (2018) UK manufacturing has lost 600,000 jobs in a decade, says Union. The Guardian. Online. Available at: https://www.theguardian.com/business/2018/jun/04/uk-manufacturing-has-lost-600000-jobs-in-a-decade-says-union

Gorz, A. (1999) *Reclaiming Work: Beyond the Wage-Based Society*. Cambridge: Polity.

Green, F. (2001) It's been a hard day's night: The concentration and intensification of work in the late twentieth-century Britain. *British Journal of Industrial Relations*, **39**, 55–80.

LexisNexis (2015) Report on the GIG economy. Online. Available at: http://lexisnexis.co.uk/pdf/Gig%20economy%20report%20-%20FINAL.pdf

Lipsedge, M., and Calnan, M. (2010) Work, stress and sickness absences psychosocial perspective. In: Baxter, P., Aw. T., Cockcroft, A., Durrington, P., and Harrington, J. (eds) *Hunters Diseases of Occupation*. 10th edn. London: Hodder Arnold, 804–22.

Mann, A., and Huddleston, P. (2017) Schools and the twenty-first century labour market: Perspectives on structural change. *British Journal of Guidance and Counselling*, **45**, 208–18.

McIvor, A. (2013) *Working Lives: Working Britain Since 1945*. Basingstoke: Belgrave.

McNair, S. (2006) How different is the older labour market? Attitudes to work and retirement among older people in Britain. *Social Policy and Society*, **5**, 485–94.

Mireia, J., Vanroelen, C., Bosmans, K., Van Aerden, K., and **Benach, J.** (2017) Precarious employment and quality of employment in relation to health and well-being in Europe. *International Journal of Health Services*, **47**, 389–409.

Noon, M., and **Blyton, P.** (2002) *The Realities of Work*. London: Palgrave.

Office of National Statistics. (2016) Women shoulder the responsibility of unpaid work. Online. Available at: https://www.ons.gov.uk/employmentandlabourmarket/peopleinwork/earningsandworkinghours/articles/womenshouldertheresponsibilityofunpaidwork/2016-11-10 [Accessed 1st July 2018].

Office of National Statistics. (2017) Graduates in the Labour Market Office, Online. Available at: https://www.ons.gov.uk/releases/graduatesintheuklabourmarket2017

Pilgrim, D. (2014) *Key Concepts in Mental Health*. 3rd edn. Thousand Oaks: Sage.

Ross, J. (2012) The current state of vocational rehabilitation services. In: Vickerstaff, S., Phillipson, C., and Wilkie, R. (eds) *Work, Health and Well-Being*. Bristol: Policy Press, 95–118.

Sennett, R. (1998) *The Corrosion of Character: The Personal Consequences of Work in the New Capitalism*. London: Norton.

Sennett, R. (2006) *The Culture of the New Capitalism*. New Haven: Yale University Press.

Standing, G. (2011) *The Precariat: The New Dangerous Class*. London: Bloomsbury.

Strangleman, T. (2007) The nostalgia for permanence at work? The end of work and its commentators. *Sociological Review*, **55**, 81–103.

Strangleman, T., and **Warren, T.** (2007) *Work and Society: Sociological Approaches, Themes and Methods*. Abingdon: Routledge.

Vickerstaff, S. (2010) The unavoidable obligation of extending our working lives? *Sociology Compass*, **4**, 869–79.

Volti, R. (2012) *An Introduction to the Sociology of Work and Occupations*. 2nd edn. London: Sage.

Wainwright, D., and **Calnan, M.** (2002) *Work Stress: The Making of a Modern Epidemic*. Buckingham: Open University Press.

Wainwright, D., and **Calnan, M.** (2012) The fall of work stress and the rise of well-being. In: Vickerstaff, S., Phillipson, C., and Wilkie, R. (eds) *Work Health and Well-being*. Bristol: Policy Press, 161–86.

Wilde, J. (2016) Precarious gigs are a perfect storm for occupational health. Online. Available at: https://www.healthandsafetyatwork.com/viewpoint/precarious-gigs-perfect-storm

Chapter 3

Chronic pain across the life span

Elaine Wainwright

Introduction

This chapter reviews the nature of pain, discussing the questions: when does pain occur and for how long, how is it thought about, how can we and should we think about it, and how does it relate to work? This includes a description of the epidemiology with a focus on the interference caused by pain and the evidence for the impact of pain across the life span.

What is pain and how do we think about it?

The word is emotive. Such a short word for a complex, affecting, powerful phenomenon. We are born in pain and may die in pain. Many humans will do a lot to avoid pain whilst also accepting that it may well be part of their lives at some point. And whilst we often think about people trying to distract themselves from their pain, pain can sometimes be looked for, even welcomed, particularly if it has an endpoint. One can think of scarification rituals, childbirth, or running races, in which pain is expected, perhaps even welcomed. Here, pain may be a key part of the process of gaining acceptance into the community, or a healthy child, or a record-beating race time (see Eccleston (2016) for great insight into the function and meaning of pain when running marathons). However, when pain is ongoing, with no end in sight, then it can have profoundly negative consequences, including disability, dysphoria, and depression. It may even provoke feelings that dying might be preferable to living with ongoing pain.

Pain may be highly threatening to our identity (Tabor et al., 2017). Pain is usually correlated in our language and our experience with suffering and loss. These phenomena occur within the individual who may struggle physically and psychologically to the extent that pain dominates their identity. Suffering and loss may also occur at the societal level, in terms of health-care costs, pain-related work absence, and health-related benefit bills (Eccleston et al., 2017). It behoves us as a society, in terms of our priorities and policies, and also as individuals responding to others, to try to reduce the suffering caused by pain. Indeed, pain relief is now recognized as a fundamental human right (Declaration of Montreal, 2010).

Pain may have biological correlates such as a slipped disc, and there are instruments like the McGill Pain Questionnaire (Melzack, 1975) which aim to capture pain location, intensity and quality to the best of human linguistic and interactional ability. However, it can be argued that there is no truly objective measure for pain; it is a subjective, embodied experience (Eccleston, 2018; Williams and Craig, 2016). People's responses to pain, as sufferer and would-be helper of the sufferer, are influenced by demographic and socioeconomic factors such as sex, gender, age, and socio-economic status (see Borsook et al., 2018, for a useful review) and psychosocial variables such as the meaning attached to the pain culturally and intrapersonally. For example, when thinking about pain and work, Andersson et al. (2011) showed an individual's risk of being sick-listed (for any condition, including pain) was higher if they had family members recently sick-listed. They suggested this may be due to an effect of social norms around sick-listing in families. Meaning is important not only for the person, influenced by their prior experience and cognitive and affective states, but also for how key stakeholders around them respond. Culturally accepted norms of suffering may be contested when pain becomes chronic. Then, observers and helpers such as health-care practitioners, family members, and employers, struggle to respond to the pained person who does not consistently improve or does not improve much at all (Wainwright et al. 2013, 2015). When thinking about pain and work, for example, it may be useful to adopt a biopsychosocial approach to considering how a relationship between the two is mediated by consciousness.

Approaches to defining pain

We can already see how complex it is to define what constitutes pain and any definition will be bound by the linguistic challenges of capturing a hugely complex experience. However, it is useful to have at least some common understanding of what people mean when they say they are in pain, so we can access some shared understanding of this when we try to ameliorate suffering. Pain is often broadly divided for medical management into acute and chronic (see Eccleston, 2016, and IASP, 2011, for useful explanations of pain terms). Acute pain lasts a relatively short time (although may be excruciating), from moments up to 3 months, and often occurs after tissue injury or nociception. Chronic pain lasts 3 months or more and may be present all the time or may fluctuate. It can be due to clearly defined causes, which may be disease related, such as rheumatoid arthritis, or may be due to a non-disease related condition, such as a slipped disc. However, chronic pain may have no clearly associated biological pathology, for example if someone suffers from ongoing back pain although no physical reason for this pain can be found. The acute–chronic distinction is a key part of clinical practice. The kind of palliative care needed in later or end of life can usefully be thought of as a third key element of clinical pain management. We may also usefully distinguish between neuropathic and nociceptive pain. The International Association for the Study of Pain (IASP) defines neuropathic pain as 'caused by a lesion or disease of the somatosensory system' (IASP, 2011) and contrasts this against nociceptive pain in which the somatosensory system is functioning normally, but pain arises from 'actual or threatened damage to non-neural tissue and is due to the activation of nociceptors' (IASP, 2011). In lay terms, nociceptive pain may be associated with tissue damage and neuropathic with nerve damage. Both can be chronic although nociceptive may be more likely to be acute; cancer pain may be nociceptive or neuropathic.

The ability to respond to acute pain throughout our lifetime can be life-saving, such as the common example of taking your hand away from a hot stove. Some short-lived pain episodes may be a normal part of growing up such as when pre-schoolers experience the scraped knees of ordinary childhood adventures. These experiences may or may not even be classed as painful by children. Other kinds of acute pain are obviously far more problematic, for example, post-surgical pain, which can now be controlled better than ever before in purely technical terms but still can be extremely challenging. This is so especially in poorly resourced settings but can be the case even in well-resourced ones. Chronic pain does not tend to have any outwardly useful function and in this important respect it is quite different from acute pain events.

IASP offered a classic definition of pain in 1979, which was carefully thought out and designed to capture the complexity of the pain experience whilst remaining practical. IASP suggested we could usefully think of pain as 'an unpleasant sensory and emotional experience associated with actual and potential tissue damage, or described in terms of such damage'. Chronic pain was defined by them as 'pain that persists beyond the normal time of healing' (IASP, 1986); compare the International Classification of Diseases-11 (ICD-11) definition of 'persistent or chronic pain lasting longer than three months' (Treede et al., 2015). These definitions have been well used and cited in the years since their publication. The IASP definitions have been praised for encompassing the multidimensional nature of pain in which, for example, there may be 'actual' tissue damage which can be identified, or concerns about potential tissue damage as described by the sufferer. The latter part of the first IASP definition, 'or described in terms of such damage' acknowledges that there may be no objective biologically determined reason for the pain, or measure for the pain, in a particular situation. Many research studies report patients struggling for validity in the face of a lack of observable pathology and also grappling with language in order to try to communicate the nature and effect of pain on their work and lives (e.g. see Johansson et al., 1999; Reid et al., 1991).The famous dictum 'pain is what the patient says it is' (Meinhart and McCaffery, 1983) asserts the patient's privilege of subjectivity so that health-care professionals must abide by what the patient says (and also by what they do to show their pain). However, some, such as phenomenological philosopher Merleau-Ponty (1962), argue that pain cannot easily be retained in consciousness. This makes it hard for some people to communicate the extent of their problems to health-care practitioners, loved ones, employers, and other stakeholders if their chronic pain condition fluctuates and happens to be waning at the time they wish to communicate with others. Additionally, as noted by Cohen and colleagues in 2018, people in pain often use metaphorical language to try to explain their pain experiences whereas health-care practitioners may use biomedical language which often has inbuilt expectations of strong relationships between tissue damage and pain reports. This leads to tension between patients who want the story of their pain to be centralized before the pain is successfully managed, and health-care practitioners who want to help but may not be able to discuss and treat the pain how the patient wishes them to. There is a huge body of literature exploring the resulting stigma some chronic pain patients feel (e.g. see McParland et al., 2011, Wainwright et al., 2015).

How else can we think about pain?

The IASP pain definition has been the subject of much debate and discussion in the past few years, as we understand more about technical aspects of how we experience pain and try to encapsulate our advanced understanding in language. Eminent pain researchers Williams and Craig recently suggested that the IASP definition underplays the seriousness of the often awful sequelae resulting from suffering with ongoing pain, as well as what we now know about the social and cognitive aspects of the pain experience. They suggest 'pain is a distressing experience associated with actual or potential tissue damage with sensory, emotional, cognitive, and social components' (Williams and Craig, 2016, p. 2420). We return to this definition below.

Cohen and colleagues argue that whilst the IASP definition has been useful, focusing our minds on the need to consider pain seriously as a mechanism for suffering, and as a clinical and public health issue, it is too narrow. They detail many reasons for this, and three of their key points, pertinent for our current consideration in this chapter—how *do* we, and how *can* we think about pain?—are as follows. First, the IASP formulation still does not release us from mind–body dualism, since this is inherent in the definition which suggests that pain may be bodily real due to actual tissue damage or 'in the mind' if tissue damage is not present. Second, Cohen and colleagues dislike the association between a pain experience and tissue damage, as there many other reasons why pain may occur, and third, they object to the singularity of ascribing a common phenomenology of 'unpleasant sensory and emotional experience' to pain. The McGill Pain Questionnaire is useful to think about here, in terms of its very wide-ranging adjectives a patient can choose from in seeking to tie down their pain in a way that could be mutually understood by them and an observer (often a health-care professional). Such adjectives include dull, sharp, spreading, and pinching (Melzack, 1975). However, this questionnaire also exemplifies how hard it may be to describe pain in the intersubjective space opened up between the person experiencing it and the person to whom they need to communicate their pain experience. In the questionnaire, patients can choose if the pain is 'radiating' and or 'spreading'. These words are not synonymous medically although they are sometimes used synonymously in the vernacular; 'pain is what the patient says it is' puts the onus on the patient to articulate in ways that may not always be achievable. If the patient is literally 'saying', then the IASP definition and McGill pain questionnaire may privilege those who are articulate. There is, of course, a critical role to be played by pain behaviours, such as guarding and holding, as part of communicating pain (see Prkachin et al., 2007), but these may also be dependent on how physically 'articulate' the pain sufferer is. Neither the IASP definition, nor that suggested by Williams and Craig, nor pain behaviour assessment, can fully solve the tension between the person in pain and the observer, if judgements about the pain experience are different. This tension may be important not only to keep social relations going but for very practical reasons such as being medically certified as able or not able to work, drive, or do some other activity, or to receive health-related sickness benefits.

Cohen and colleagues propose a new definition which they suggest can ameliorate the tension between the privileging of self-report against the dependency on the observer to judge the qualities of the pain experience. They wish this to apply to clinical situations. They also seek to move from 'damage' to 'threat' since this may be more in line with modern non-judgemental conceptualizations that there may be no identifiable physical damage yet the pain is threatening the person's nature and integrity. They propose 'pain is a mutually recognisable somatic experience that reflects a person's apprehension of threat to their bodily or existential integrity' (Cohen et al., p. 6). The authors write that the 'mutually recognisable' part of their definition should enable 'a clinical encounter that ensures a mutual exploration of the patient's beliefs, expectations and perceived meanings of pain' (p. 6) and one hopes it will. However, consider, for example, the eyeballing of one particular doctor and one particular patient, when the patient seeks either to be, or not to be, certified as having workability, in a sickness certification consultation. It is hard to see here how changing the definition alone will reduce pain's ability to disrupt the doctor–patient relationship when we know doctors may dislike certifying for pain since it can be hard to map its subjectivity onto specific workability requirements. Still, in time, the linguistic change may encourage behaviour change towards a more mutual recognition of the pain and its impacts.

The word 'somatic' may be useful since it removes the dichotomous idea that pain is in the body *or* the mind and locates it in the body. A related yet different conceptualization of the relationship between the body and the pain experience is that it is 'embodied', as put forward by Tabor and colleagues in 2017 and Eccleston in 2018. Tabor et al. write compellingly of the importance of emphasizing that the body is 'not separate from the brain nor the world, but part of the facility that actively shapes our experience of pain' (p. 1007). They show how this way of seeing pain defines it 'in terms of action: an experience that, as part of a protective strategy, attempts to defend one's *self* in the presence of inferred threat' (p. 1007, [emphasis in the original]). This definition is part of modern movements to approach pain from a motivational perspective, as pain here is always about action. Chronic pain evokes ongoing actions to try to reduce the persistent threat of pain that is not ending. One can immediately see how this is exhausting for the sufferer. Taking the conceptualizion of chronic pain as embodied defence further, Eccleston (2018) argues we must reposition pain as 'always and inescapably an urge to return the organism to coherence, as always acting in and on the world, and as always functioning to protect from predicted harm' (p. S17). This embodied pain framework highlights pain as defending against harm and promoting behavioural coherence. The embodied view of pain as an action against uncertainty and threat means that if we are to reduce pain intrusion and interference (including whilst we work, or more broadly occupy ourselves) we must attend more deeply to how people manage threats to identity and coherence.

To summarise this chapter so far, pain can be thought about at individual, social, and global levels and discursively defined in different ontological and epistemological ways. There is no absolute agreement on how to think about it and define it at present. However, there are movements to bridge the sufferer–observer, subjective–objective gap, and to think about pain from a functional perspective as opposed to conceptualizing it simply as an experience. How pain is thought about, and defined, has important implications for clinical, research, and policy agendas. We need these agendas to seek better relief from pain than we achieve today.

The epidemiology of pain

The definitions of pain presented here could be applied to a vast range of symptoms and conditions, including backache, headaches, and persistent or recurring pain in any part of the body. This broad application can be useful and also makes it very difficult to know exactly how many people suffer from pain conditions. Goldberg and McGee (2011) show that the four largest causes of pain are cancer, osteo- and rheumatoid arthritis, operations and injuries, and spinal problems, making pain aetiology very complex. To complicate how we define and collect data about pain further, we know that there are high rates of co-morbidity between pain and other conditions, such as depression. For example, in a landmark survey of 15 European countries and Israel, Breivik et al. (2006) found that 21% of chronic pain patients were depressed because of their pain.

Despite the complexity of what is 'pain', most researchers use the IASP or ICD-11 definitions and argue that we must try to reduce the burden of pain. Returning to our young students scraping their knees, whilst the knee scrape itself may be a normal developmental experience, there are data showing that for some children, notably when they reach adolescence and also particularly for girls, pain does becomes chronic and problematic. A review found that headache, abdominal and back pain were the largest problems, with, for example, 8–83% of populations surveyed reporting ongoing headache pain was an issue (King et al., 2011). Prevalence rates varied dramatically between studies, and there were quality issues with the original studies, but the extent of chronic pain reported was worrying. Palermo and colleagues (2014) point out that many epidemiological studies report prevalence, not pain severity or impact; there is a subset of young people with chronic pain who do experience moderate to severe disability who need targeted help.

When considering adults, we know that pain, and particularly chronic pain, is one of the most significant health burdens of our time. Goldberg and McGee (2011) make a powerful case for viewing pain as a global public health priority, based on its 'staggering prevalence' (p.2). They argue that whilst it can be hard to quantify pain, due to its fluctuating and multifactorial nature, the best evidence we have estimates that 20% of adults globally suffer from pain and 10% are newly diagnosed with chronic pain per year. They cite evidence that primary care settings in Africa, the Americas, Asia, and Europe find patients reporting persistent pain prevalence of 10–35%. Jackson et al. (2015) estimated 33% of the adult population in lower and middle-income countries is affected by chronic pain.

A milestone survey found that one in five Europeans has chronic pain which has lasted 6 months or more, occurs frequently or is even present most of the time, and is severe in its intensity (Breivik et al., 2006). More recently, Breivik and colleagues reviewed population-based surveys in many different European countries and found these consistently estimate that between 24–35% of adults report chronic pain (Breivik et al., 2013). Part of the difference in these percentages is due to different ways in which we can define and collect data about who is suffering with pain. Similar prevalence rates and ranges are found in other studies e.g. a meta-analysis by Fayaz et al. (2016) estimated a prevalence rate of 35.0–51.3% for the UK.

There are many documented risk factors for developing chronic pain after an acute pain event, including lifestyle factors, tendency towards negative affect, age, being female, low socio-economic status, and tissue injury via accidents or surgery (see Breivik, 2017, for a comprehensive overview).

Anyone can experience pain; notably cancer pain is present in settings with access to the best resources; see work by Breivik and colleagues (2009) and Foley (2011). However, the pain burden is not distributed equally around the world. Goldberg and McGee (2011) explain how those who are most disadvantaged (and usually living in the south of the world) suffer the global pain burden more than those in the north, and also tend to have access to poorer treatment regimes. There are clearly issues of ethics and social justice at play here since we should work towards pain relief as a human right for all.

The impact of pain

The impact of pain across the life span can be terrible. This chapter specifically considers the impact on paid work below. Briefly, the broader impact can include loss of schooling, happiness, physical functioning, relationships, and sense of a coherent self. For example, children and young people in pain appear to show more challenging temperaments than peers and are also more sensitive to pain (Palermo et al., 2014). Studies have shown that parenting a child with pain is difficult, involving greater financial outlay and social restrictions on family life (see Eccleston et al., 2004; Sleed et al., 2005 and the discussion of parenting in Chapter 4).

Less is known about the impact of pain on the transitional years between adolescence and adulthood (taken up in Chapters 5 and 6) or in later life production (see Chapter 8), but there are hundreds of studies demonstrating the impact on adult life. Ongoing pain is often co-morbid with psychological disorders, and this combination can lead to substantial impairment of day-to-day activities and relationships for people around the world (Gureje et al., 2001). There are huge financial and psychosocial costs to the pain patient, including not being able to get work or keep it, stigma from societal views of people who do not get better, and (if one is lucky enough to live in a system that offers care) travelling to appointments, as well as the equipment and medication needed to manage one's pain. The cost to society is also enormous, and, depending on individual countries' workplace and welfare systems, can include productivity losses, health-related benefits, the cost of health services themselves, and so on. We now turn to an overview of how pain impacts on work.

How does pain impact on work?

We know that pain has substantial deleterious effects on work. Studies which examine this are many, although few look at work outside paid full or part-time jobs, as opposed to the broader sense of occupation used in this book, which may include parenting, schooling or voluntary work. Chapter 4 debates parenting and pain, and Chapter 5, schooling. There is also little known about the impact of pain on occupation in a broad sense for those in transition between the teenage years and post-school working life. Little is known about the effects of pain on undertaking voluntary work. A few studies do show that voluntary work may ameliorate pain effects. In 2002, Arnstein and colleagues found pain intensity scores dropped after volunteering and in 2017, Salt and colleagues reported that volunteering had a role in improving life purpose for women in pain.

Most research regarding pain impact on work looks at paid work and reduction in work participation linked to people's pain. However, even narrowing our focus thus, many studies do not look at the quality of the work which people might want to secure. It may be that not all the work studied is 'safe and appropriate', to use the seminal phrase coined by Waddell and Burton (2006), but is, rather, a necessity, even if there are other risk factors attendant, such as work-related burnout. It may be that even if the work itself in these studies would not be classed as 'good', the worker requires it, for financial, social, or other reasons. Studies tend to record basic work characteristics, such as whether the job includes manual labour, the sector, and the level studied (e.g. telling readers we are looking at junior nurses within a hospital in a certain city), but often do not say much about whether there are any known associated job strains or satisfactions with the particular workplaces being studied or the role per se. For example, studies of nurses might not tell us, or might not ascertain, if the particular nurses studied are concerned by a poorly regulated shift pattern in their location, or whether changing societal attitudes to medics are affecting how they feel about, perhaps even how they do, their jobs. There is also a growing body of research that is beginning to understand the fine grain of how pain interferes with attention that we may need to consider when thinking about how pain impacts on work. For example, Attridge et al. (2017) found that headache pain slows people down relative to when they are headache free in multiple attention tasks, mostly those involving attentional switching or selective attention. This might be important if we think about the pain impact on particular workplace tasks. It also might be important as part of broader research into what kinds of work tasks might help to reduce the impact of pain. All these things might matter if we are thinking about how best to enable people in pain to achieve sustainable 'safe and appropriate' working lives. Even if we do not know much about these things, study participants seem to want to work, or they have to, and we do know a lot about the macro impacts of pain on paid work, such as absenteeism and presenteeism, briefly exemplified below.

Almost 20% of participants with chronic pain surveyed by Breivik et al. (2006) said that they had lost their job due to their pain condition, and 33% stated that the time they could work, indeed whether they were able to work at all, was affected by their chronic pain. In 2013, Breivik and colleagues discussed recent studies showing that that at least half of those with chronic pain stated that it interfered with their work. A systematic review of observational studies reported that chronic pain has substantial deleterious effects on work absenteeism and presenteeism across Europe (Patel et al., 2012). For example, of 37 studies that considered associations between chronic pain and employment status, 35 reported pain had a negative impact. Interference in employment due to pain was reported in 26% to 88% of participants. Langley and colleagues (2013) found that neuropathic pain may have a particularly severe impact on work, since neuropathic pain sufferers had lower rates of labour force participation and higher absenteeism and presenteeism relative to a chronic pain reference group.

Musculoskeletal (MSK) disorders are the second most frequent reason for being sick-listed in the UK primary care system (after mental health problems), accounting for approximately 20% of certificates (Wynne-Jones et al., 2010). In 2017/18, 6.6 million working days were lost due to work-related MSK disorders in the UK (HSE, 2018). Back pain is estimated to cost the UK economy £12.3 billion per annum (Bevan, 2016). In Finland, it has been found that chronic pain accounts for nearly 30% of medically certified absence lasting more than a fortnight (Saastamoinen et al., 2009). This has clear personal and financial implications for patients.

A recent systematic review and meta-analysis examined absence from work and return-to-work in people with back pain in cohort studies (Wynne-Jones et al., 2014). The authors pointed out that prospective studies in workers with back pain vary in setting and design, thus aimed to provide a quantitative summary of current evidence. The pooled estimate for the proportion of people with back pain returning to work was 68.2% at 1 month, 85.6% at 1–6 months, and 93.3% at ≥ 6 months. This suggests a good return-to-work rate but the 32% of people not back at 1 month are key targets, to prevent long-term absence. The authors also stated that differences in setting and methods of ascertaining work absence explained some of the variation.

So, what can we do to help people in pain return to, or stay at, work? Section three of this book, Interventions, analyses this question in detail, from psychological, policy-making, and multidisciplinary interventionist perspectives. Briefly, here, it is useful to note that there are interventions which work, but many meta-analyses show that key elements of trials (e.g. populations, interventions, comparators, outcomes) can be hard to compare due to heterogeneity. Some recent, important research findings are summarized below.

Two recent systematic reviews and meta-analyses do not make for comforting reading. Pike et al. (2016) reviewed the effectiveness of psychological interventions for chronic pain on health-care use and work absence. They found that there were no significant effects of psychological interventions over comparison on work loss but that a summary was challenging, as studies used so many different measures. Cochrane et al. (2017) reviewed early interventions to promote work participation in people with regional MSK pain. This included trials if they reported on work-based outcomes for participants experiencing difficulties at work or ≤ 3-months' sick leave. Interventions had to include two or more elements of the biopsychosocial model delivered as a co-ordinated programme. They found that at 12-months' follow-up, there was moderate quality evidence to suggest that programmes involving a stepped care approach were more effective than the comparisons in promoting return-to-work (hazard ratio (HR) 1.29 (95% confidence interval (CI) 1.03 to 1.61), $p = 0.03$), whereas case management was not (HR 0.92 (95% CI 0.69 to 1.24), $p = 0.59$). Their analyses suggested only limited effectiveness in reducing sickness absences, in pain reduction, or functional improvement across the intervention categories. They concluded that there was uncertainty as to the effectiveness of early multicomponent interventions owing to clinical and insurance system heterogeneity.

More promisingly, Cullen et al. (2017) examined effectiveness of workplace-based return-to-work interventions and work disability management interventions that assist workers with MSK and pain-related conditions and mental health conditions. They found strong evidence that duration away from work from both MSK or pain-related conditions and mental health conditions was significantly reduced by multidomain interventions encompassing at least two of their three target domains (health-focused, service coordination, and work modification interventions).

In summary, pain impacts on the quality and quantity of work that people living with it can do. There are some promising interventions that may ameliorate the effects of pain. As we learn more about exactly what kinds of pain have what kinds of effects on work, and on different types of work, we should plan to incorporate this knowledge into intervention design and also into how we think about, and might design, work. If work is to be a yardstick by which we measure an individual's worth, for example, then we need to give that individual the best chance of making a good contribution, with or without pain.

Summary

We do not have complete agreement amongst people living with pain, researchers, practitioners, and policy-makers regarding how we think about, and define, pain. However, many stakeholders agree we can see it at different discursive levels: as an individual tragedy, as an important societal issue, and as a potentially disastrous public health issue.

Modern ways of thinking about pain focus on its embodied nature, and its extant function in protecting the organism from threat.

The epidemiology of pain shows an enormous burden of ill-health globally in terms of prevalence, and costs to society through use of health care, uptake of health-related incapacity benefits, and the suffering of the populace.

Research into the impact of pain shows it can affect almost every facet of psychological and physical functioning for an individual, with far-reaching consequences for their quality of life.

The impact of pain on paid work is substantial although we know much less about how it impacts on other forms of occupation.

These different discursive formations of how we view pain need to be encapsulated in whatever we decide as a society we can do, to reduce the pain burden on individuals. The embodied view of pain as an action against uncertainty means that if we are to reduce pain intrusion and interference (including whilst we work, or more broadly occupy ourselves) we must attend more deeply to how people manage threats to identity and coherence.

References

Andersson, F. W., Bokenblom, M., Brantingson, S. Brännström, S. G., and Wall, J. (2011) Sick-listing—Partly a family phenomenon? *Journal of Socio-Economics*, **40**, 496–502.

Arnstein, P., Vidal, M., Wells-Federman, C., Morgan, B., and Caudill, M. (2002) From chronic pain patient to peer: Benefits and risks of volunteering. *Pain Management Nursing*, **3**, 94–103.

Attridge, N., Eccleston, C., Noonan, D., Wainwright, E., and Keogh, E. (2017) Headache impairs attentional performance: A conceptual replication and extension. *The Journal of Pain*, **18**, 29–41.

Bevan, S. (2016) Workplace Health in the UK. *American Journal of Health Promotion*, **30**, 396–8.

Borsook, D., Youssef, A. M., Simons, L., Elman, I., and Eccleston, C. (2018) When pain gets stuck: The evolution of pain chronification and treatment resistance. *Pain*, **159**, 2421–36.

Breivik, H. (2017) Epidemiology of pain: its importance for clinical management and research. In: Eccleston, C., Wells, C., and Morlion, B. (eds), *European Pain Management*. Oxford: OUP, 8–16.

Breivik, H., Cherny, N., Collett, B., De Conno, F., Filbet, M., Foubert, A. J., et al. (2009) Cancer-related pain: A pan-European survey of prevalence, treatment, and patient attitudes. *Annals of Oncology*, **20**, 1420–33.

Breivik, H., Collett, B., Ventafridda, V., Cohen, R., and Gallacher, D. (2006) Survey of chronic pain in Europe: Prevalence, impact on daily life, and treatment. *European Journal of Pain*, **10**, 287–333.

Breivik, H., Eisenberg, E., and O'Brien, T. (2013) The individual and societal burden of chronic pain in Europe: the case for strategic prioritisation and action to improve knowledge and availability of appropriate care. *BMC Public Health*, **13**, 1229.

Cochrane, A., Higgins, N. M., FitzGerald, O., Gallagher, P., Ashton, J., Corcoran, O., and Desmond, D. (2017) Early interventions to promote work participation in people with regional musculoskeletal pain: a systematic review and meta-analysis. *Clinical Rehabilitation*, **31**, 1466–81.

Cohen, M., Quintner, J., and van Rysewyk, S. (2018) Reconsidering the International Association for the Study of Pain definition of pain. *Pain Reports*, **3**, e634.

Cullen, K. L., Irvin, E., Collie, A., Clay, F., Gensby, U., Jennings, P. A., et al. (2017) Effectiveness of workplace interventions in return-to-work for musculoskeletal, pain-related and mental health conditions: An update of the evidence and messages for practitioners. *Journal of Occupational Rehabilitation*, **28**, 1–15.

Declaration of Montreal. (2010) Declaration of Montreal. Online. Available at: http://www.iasp-pain.org/files/Content/NavigationMenu/Advocacy/DeclarationOfMontreal.pdf

Eccleston, C. (2016) *Embodied: the Psychology of Physical Sensation*. Oxford: Oxford University Press.

Eccleston, C. (2018) Chronic pain as embodied defence: Implications for current and future psychological treatments. *Pain*, **159** Suppl 1, S17–23.

Eccleston, C., Crombez, G., Scotford, A., Clinch, J., and Connell, H. (2004) Adolescent chronic pain: Patterns and predictors of emotional distress in adolescents with chronic pain and their parents. *Pain*, **108**, 221–9.

Eccleston, C., Wells, C., and Morlion, B. (eds) (2017) *European Pain Management*. Oxford, OUP.

Fayaz, A., Croft, P., Landford, R. M, Donaldson, L. J., Jones, G. T., et al. (2016) Prevalence of chronic pain in the UK. *BMJ Open*; **6**: e010364.

Foley, K. M. (2011) How well is cancer pain treated? *Palliative Medicine*, **25**, 398–401.

Goldberg, D., and McGee, S. (2011) Pain as a global health priority. *BMC Public Health* **11**, 770.

Gureje, O., Simon, G.E., and Von Korff, M. (2001) A cross-national study of the course of persistent pain in primary care. *Pain*, **92**, 195–200.

Health and Safety Executive, (HSE). (2018) Work related musculoskeletal disorders in Great Britain (WRMSDs), 2018. Online. Available at: http://www.hse.gov.uk/statistics/causdis/msd.pdf [Accessed 23rd July 2019]

International Association for the Study of Pain (IASP). (1979) Pain terms: A list with definitions and notes on usage: recommended by the IASP Subcommittee on Taxonomy. *Pain*, **6**, 249.

International Association for the Study of Pain (IASP) (1986) Subcommittee on Taxonomy Classification of chronic pain. Descriptions of chronic pain syndromes and definitions of pain terms. *Pain*, **3**, S1–226.

International Association for the Study of Pain (IASP). (2011) https://www.iasp-pain.org/terminology?navItemNumber=576#Neuropathicpain

Jackson, T., Thomas, S., Stabile, V., Han, X., Shotwell, M., and McQueen, K. (2015) Prevalence of chronic pain in low-income and middle-income countries: A systematic review and meta-analysis. *Lancet*, **385**(Suppl. 2): S10.

Johansson, E. E., Hamberg, K., Westman, G. and Lindgren, G. (1999) The meanings of pain: An exploration of women's descriptions of symptoms. *Social Science and Medicine*, **48**, 1791–1802.

King, S., Chambers, C. T., Huguet, A., MacNevin, R. C., McGrath, P. J., Parker, L., and MacDonald, A. J. (2011) The epidemiology of chronic pain in children and adolescents revisited: A systematic review. *Pain*, **152**, 2729–38.

Langley, P. C., Van Litsenburg, C., Cappelleri, J. C., and Carroll, D. (2013) The burden associated with neuropathic pain in Western Europe. *Journal of Medical Economics*, **16**, 85–95.

McParland, J., Eccleston, C., Osborn, M., and Hezseltine, L. (2011) It's not fair: An Interpretative Phenomenological Analysis of discourses of justice and fairness in chronic pain. *Health*, **15**, 459–74.

Meinhart, N. T., and McCaffery, M. (1983) *Pain: A Nursing Approach to Assessment and Analysis.* Norwalk, CT: Appleton-Century-Crofts.

Melzack, R. (1975) The McGill Pain Questionnaire: Major properties and scoring methods. *Pain*, **1**, 277–99.

Merleau-Ponty, M. (1962) *Phenomenology of Perception.* London: Routledge and Kegan Paul.

Palermo, T. M., Valrie, C. R., and Karlson, C. W. (2014) Family and parent influences on pediatric chronic pain: A developmental perspective. *American Psychologist*, **69**, 142–52.

Patel, A. S., Farquharson, R., Carroll, D., Moore, A., Phillips, C. J., Taylor, R. S., and Barden, J. (2012) The impact and burden of chronic pain in the workplace: A qualitative systematic review. *Pain Practice*, **12**, 578–89.

Pike, A., Hearn, L., and Williams, A. C. de C. (2016) Effectiveness of psychological interventions for chronic pain on health care use and work absence: Systematic review and meta-analysis. *Pain*, **157**, 777–85.

Prkachin, K. M., Schultz, I. Z., and Hughes, E. (2007) Pain behaviour and the development of pain-related disability: The importance of guarding. *Clinical Journal of Pain*, **23**, 270–7.

Reid, J., Ewan, C., and Lowry, E. (1991) Pilgrimage of pain: The illness experiences of women with repetitive strain injury and the search for credibility. *Social Science and Medicine*, **32**, 601–12.

Saastamoinen, P., Laaksonen, M., Lahelma, E., and Leino-Arjas, P. (2009) The effect of pain on sickness absence among middle-aged municipal employees. *Occupational and Environmental Medicine*, **66**, 131–6.

Salt, E., Crofford, L. J., and Segerstrom, S. (2017) The mediating and moderating effect of volunteering on pain and depression, life purpose, well-being, and physical activity. *Pain Management Nursing*, **18**, 243–9.

Sleed, M., Eccleston, C., Beecham, J., Knapp, M., and Jordan, A. (2005) The economic impact of chronic pain in adolescence: Methodological considerations and a preliminary costs-of-illness study. *Pain*, **119**, 183–90.

Tabor, A., Keogh, E., and Eccleston, C. (2017) Embodied pain—negotiating the boundaries of possible action. *Pain*, **158**, 1007–11.

Treede, R. D., Reif, W., Barke A, Aziz, Q., Bennett, M. I., Benoliel, R., et al. (2015) A classification of chronic pain for ICD-11. *Pain*, **156**, 1003–7.

Waddell, G., and Burton, K. (2006) *Is Work Good for Your Health and Well-being?* London: The Stationary Office.

Wainwright, E., Wainwright, D., Keogh, E., and Eccleston, C. (2013) Return to work with chronic pain: employers' and employees' views. *Occupational Medicine*, **63**, 501–6.

Wainwright, E., Wainwright, D., Keogh, E., and Eccleston, C. (2015) The social negotiation of fitness for work: Tensions in doctor–patient relationships over medical certification of chronic pain. *Health*, **19**, 17–33.

Williams, A. C., and Craig, K. D. (2016) Updating the definition of pain. *Pain*, **157**, 2420–3.

Wynne-Jones, G., Mallen, C. D., and Dunn, K. M. (2010) Sickness certification for musculoskeletal conditions. *Clinical Rheumatology* **29**, 573–4.

Wynne-Jones, G., Cowen, J., Jordan, J. L., Uthman, O., Main, C. J., Glozier, N., and van der Windt, D. (2014) Absence from work and return-to-work in people with back pain: a systematic review and meta-analysis. *Occupational and Environmental Medicine*, **71**, 448–56.

Section 2

Investigations

Chapter 4

Parenting in the context of chronic pain

Abbie Jordan and Tiina Jaaniste

Introduction

Parenting is a 'significant life-changing event and a defining feature of adult life' (Palermo and Eccleston, 2009, p. 15). Quality parenting has been defined as the ability to respond positively to the changing needs and circumstances of children (Crawford, 2011). It encompasses both meeting the basic needs of a child, such as shelter, nutrition, clothing, and health care, in addition to the process of promoting and supporting physical, emotional, social, and intellectual development from birth through to adulthood (Armstrong et al., 2005; Bornstein, 2006). Parents may choose to take primary responsibility for addressing the above needs themselves, or they may share, or outsource, some of the above roles to schools, nannies, tutors, childcare centres, grandparents, or others. In other words, parenting entails a set of roles that the parent may choose to adopt themselves or they may find another person or organization to whom they can delegate certain responsibilities, potentially in exchange of payment. In this respect parenting may be considered as work. Given that parenting spans such an extended time-frame, in most cases, parents still oversee the overall care and needs of their child and recruit various external supports at times as needed, depending on their own capacity to fulfil the various roles. Although it is common for parents to engage in paid work outside of the home as well as their parenting roles, parents who are highly engaged in parenting roles may have less capacity to engage in other occupational roles. This may be particularly true if some aspects of the parenting roles are highly challenging or time-consuming, such as meeting the needs of a child with a long-term health condition.

Parenting is widely recognized to be both rewarding and challenging. Yet, parenting a child who has chronic pain poses additional stressors and challenges for the parent. Chronic pain has the potential to interrupt or alter the 'typical' development of a child or adolescent across any number of areas of development (Eccleston et al., 2008). Parents of children with chronic pain are often unsure about how best to support their child through the myriad of normative developmental tasks, in addition to the unique challenges associated with their child's experience of pain and associated disability. This chapter will review the impact of paediatric chronic pain on parents, particularly regarding their psychological, social, and financial well-being. The complex, bidirectional relationships between paediatric chronic pain, and family relationships and attachment, will be considered. Following a brief overview of how parents may respond to their child's pain and pain behaviours, consideration will be given to why parents respond in particular ways. Specifically, the role of parental appraisal of their child's pain and pain behaviours, in addition to parental risk and resilience factors, will be reviewed. The chapter will also briefly consider parenting in the context of living with parental chronic pain. Implications for best clinical practice and future research directions will be discussed.

Parental impact and experience in the context of paediatric pain

Parenting a child with chronic pain is inherently stressful (Darlington et al., 2011; Eccleston et al., 2004). Unsurprisingly, the highest levels of parenting stress are reported by parents of youth with the greatest levels of pain-related disability (Cohen et al., 2010). Mothers of youth with chronic pain also report significantly elevated levels of anxiety and depression compared with mothers of youth without chronic pain (Campo et al., 2007). For numerous parents of youth with chronic pain, levels of anxiety and depression reach or exceed clinically significant levels (Eccleston et al., 2004). Studies have begun to explore additional mental health symptomatology. One study found that 9% of parents of youth with chronic pain reported post-traumatic stress disorder (PTSD) symptoms at clinically significant levels (Neville et al., 2018). Interestingly, parental PTSD symptoms in this study were typically related to the child's pain outcomes such as pain interference, rather than being a separate yet co-occurring entity.

Studies have demonstrated that parents are distressed by the sense of helplessness they experience due to their inability to relieve their child's pain. For some parents, this powerlessness to 'make things better' may result in a perceived loss of role as a protector for their child and a need to re-conceptualize ways in which to parent their child (Jordan et al., 2007; Jordan et al., 2016; Maciver et al., 2010).

The effects of parenting a child or adolescent with chronic pain are broad, affecting parental social and physical functioning. Parents of youth with long-term health conditions (including pain-specific conditions) report substantial reductions in the amount and quality of sleep due to night-time caregiving requirements, illness monitoring, and parenting stress (Meltzer and Moore, 2008). Additionally, parents of youth with chronic pain report poorer health-related quality of life (Mano et al., 2011) and social restriction. In particular, parents of youth with chronic pain report a restricted ability to engage with social activities, in part related to an ever-present need to be on call for their child (Hunfeld et al., 2001; Jordan et al., 2007).

Importantly, most of the parenting studies in this literature have predominantly involved mothers. However, fathers are also likely to be impacted by their child's chronic pain and associated disability. Much less is known about the experience of fathers in the context of having a child with chronic pain; however, some differences have been noted. Mothers of children with rheumatic disease have been found to report significantly higher levels of depressed mood compared with fathers (Timko et al., 1992). Similarly, mothers of youth with chronic pain report significantly lower levels of health-related quality of life and higher levels of catastrophizing respectively, compared with fathers (Hechler et al., 2011; Mano et al., 2011).

Whilst the literature suggests a more negative and pervasive impact of chronic paediatric pain on mothers, one study identified a unique focus on re-evaluation of relationships with their adolescent experiencing pain for fathers. In a unique paternally focused study, fathers reported a need to re-evaluate their relationships with their adolescent children due to no longer being able to engage with shared activities as a result of pain (Jordan et al., 2016). For some fathers, this re-evaluation resulted in a weakening of the relationship with their child, yet other fathers described a strengthening of their relationship due to a new focus on quality of life rather than shared physical activities. Broadly, these varied results may, in part, stem from differences in the roles that mothers and fathers have, with mothers often spending more time with their child and having a greater role in the everyday management of their child's pain.

Costs of paediatric chronic pain

In clinical encounters, parents anecdotally comment about the financial burden associated with their child's chronic pain. Although there have been some analyses of the costs associated with paediatric chronic pain, particularly with respect to costs associated with interdisciplinary treatment programmes (Mahrer et al., 2018), less is known about the direct and indirect costs borne by parents. One US study found that out of pocket costs for parents totalled $3319, with additional costs ascribed to employing extra help, transport, special equipment, and special food and supplements (Groenewald et al., 2014). Notably, informal care costs were high in this study, with parents paying for an average of 343 hours of informal care per adolescent each year. Similar costs for parents of adolescents with chronic pain were identified in a smaller UK study, with total out of pocket costs estimated at £900 per family per year (Sleed et al., 2005).

Other sources of indirect costs for parents of youth with chronic pain are related to work absences and reduced productivity. Days absent from work due to responsibilities associated with caring for a dependent with chronic pain are commonly reported. Estimations of number of lost working days for parents vary across studies ranging from 7 to 37 days per family each year (Groenewald et al., 2014; Sleed et al., 2005). Interestingly, a higher number of days absent from work are reported by parents who report low confidence in their child's ability to cope with the pain, even when controlling for the child's level of functioning (Jaaniste et al., 2016). Although findings are compelling, it is important to be mindful that cost-related studies have typically focused on exploring costs in small samples of families with youth with high levels of pain-related disability, posing issues in terms of generalizability of findings (Groenewald and Palermo, 2015).

Whilst work absence costs have financial implications at an individual level, the potential implications are wider reaching for parents in terms of employment and missed opportunities. For example, a minority of parents reported having to give up work altogether or moving to lower paid, more flexible roles to meet caregiving demands associated with parenting a child with chronic pain (Groenewald et al., 2014; Ho et al.,

2008; Sleed et al., 2005). Such decisions may result in reduced career opportunities for parents, both in the short and long term. For example, reducing hours may result in a parent being unable to take on additional roles, resulting in an increased time period until promotion. Resigning from an existing role due to caregiving needs may result in a desired career no longer being viable.

Despite the substantial personal and societal financial 'cost' implications associated with reduced parental engagement in the workplace as a result of parenting a child with chronic pain, there is a dearth of research in this particular area. In particular, nothing is known concerning how difficult decisions around engagement with employment is associated with parental well-being and functioning.

Parenting in the context of living with chronic pain

Although discussion has focused on the experiences of parents in the context of parenting a child or adolescent with chronic pain, it is important to acknowledge that parents themselves may experience chronic pain. The adult epidemiological literature identifies an increase in the prevalence of chronic pain across the adult age span (Fayaz et al., 2016), and a sizeable number of adults with chronic pain are themselves parents. Yet, little is known about how parents who experience chronic pain simultaneously manage the physically and psychologically demanding tasks of parenting.

Mothers with chronic pain report significantly impaired psychological, physical, and familial functioning compared with mothers without chronic pain, with the largest number of parenting challenges reported by mothers with the most impaired psychological functioning (Evans et al., 2005). Such challenges include difficulties with providing physical comfort to children, facilitating their child's engagement in social activities, in addition to attending school and sports events (Evans and de Souza, 2008; Umberger and Risko, 2016). These activities, of course, reflect part of the 'work' of parenting.

Recent work in this area has addressed parents' perceptions of challenges associated with parenting in the context of living with a chronic pain condition (Wilson and Fales, 2016). Findings identified that an overwhelming 86% of parents reported reduced parental involvement, with a notable, although smaller, percentage reporting more inconsistent discipline practices and increased impatience with their adolescents due to their own pain. Interestingly, though, studies which elicited the retrospective reflections of adolescents regarding living with a parent with chronic pain, identified positive aspects of the adolescents' experiences, such as the development of valuable life skills as a result of adopting additional responsibilities (Umberger and Risko, 2016). Such findings highlight the complexity of this issue and the importance of considering time points at which reports are elicited.

It should be acknowledged that children of parents with chronic pain are more likely to develop chronic pain than children of parents without chronic pain (McKillop and Banez, 2016). In addition to the potential role of genetic factors, another suggested mechanism for this transmission is parental modelling of pain behaviours, with parental modelling showing a stronger relationship with adolescent self-reported pain severity and impairment than parental response behaviours to their adolescent's pain (Stone et al., 2018).

How chronic pain impacts on family dynamics and the role of parent–child attachment

Although chronic pain is a personal, individual experience, it occurs within a broader social context (Craig, 2009; Craig, 2015). One systematic review reported poorer family functioning of children and adolescents with chronic pain compared with healthy controls in five out of seven studies (Lewandowski et al., 2010). Moreover, in six of the nine studies, greater child disability was associated with poorer family functioning. However, all reviewed studies were cross-sectional, making it impossible to establish direction of causality. It may be that the child's pain experience leads to heightened family stress and, consequently, poorer family functioning. Alternatively, families who are functioning poorly may be more likely to have children who subsequently develop and maintain problems such as chronic pain, perhaps due to poorer coping resources (Minuchin et al., 1975).

In the early years of life, the parent–child relationship is typically the most important aspect of a child's social environment. It has been suggested that early parent–child attachment patterns may form a template for future relationships (Malekpour, 2007). Despite the early development and relative stability of attachment styles, they are nevertheless changeable (Hamilton, 2000). Negative life experiences have been found to be a significant predictor of change in a child's attachment classification between infancy and adolescence (Hamilton, 2000). Paediatric chronic pain is a significant stressor with a strong psycho-social component and thus may lead to significant changes in parent–child relationships. However, research is lacking in this area.

Given that attachment behaviours may be conceptualized as behaviours that promote safety (Crittenden, 1999), the development of chronic pain may result in a new set of principles guiding both child and parent behaviour as they strive to avoid pain (Donnelly and Jaaniste, 2016). These new guiding principles may become so strong that they override other previously valued principles, guiding behaviour, and governing attention. For example, despite a parent's previous support of their adolescent's growing autonomy, this goal may be disregarded if the parent perceives it to contradict the more dominant desire to promote their child's safety and avoidance of pain.

How a parent responds to their child's chronic pain

How a parent responds to their child's chronic pain may have a significant impact on the child's functioning and hence their maintenance or recovery from pain. Parents generally want the best for their child; however, well-intended responses to their child's pain and associated behaviours are sometimes unhelpful. Miscarried helping can occur when a parent's desire to be helpful inadvertently contributes to negative parent–child interactions regarding health behaviours, which may result in poorer pain and functional outcomes over time (Fales et al., 2014).

Helpful and unhelpful parental responses to a child's chronic pain have traditionally been considered within an operant paradigm (e.g. reinforcing adaptive behaviours, discouraging maladaptive behaviours) (Lewandowski et al., 2010). A detailed review of specific parental behaviours and attitudes in response to child pain is beyond the scope of this chapter. However, Table 4.1 summarizes the key parental behaviours and attitudes which have been studied in the literature. The overall helpfulness of the behaviour or attitude is noted; however, it should be acknowledged that child individual difference factors may moderate the impact of some parental responses.

More recently, there has been a call for greater recognition of the bi-directional influences between the parent and child within the paediatric chronic pain context (e.g. Lewandowski et al., 2010), resulting in the development of new approaches for dyadic research. The Actor–Partner Interdependence Model (APIM; Cook and Kenny, 2005) is a longitudinal model for assessing bi-directional effects in relationships, and has been effectively applied to the study of child–parent interactions within a pain context (Birnie et al., 2016; Birnie et al., 2017; Fales et al., 2014).

Factors that influence parental response to their child's chronic pain

When individuals are faced with stressors, ways in which they respond will be influenced by a broad array of inter-related factors. Stable personality factors, such as trait anxiety and empathy, may influence parental response to stressful situations. Parental appraisal of the problem and of their own capacity to respond will also influence their response. Furthermore, a range of parental resilience and risk factors may contribute to how parents respond to stressors. These factors will be reviewed and considered in the context of how parents respond to their child's pain and pain behaviours.

Parental personality and response to their child's pain

Personality refers to stable individual differences in characteristic patterns of thinking, feeling, and behaving that determine how an individual adjusts to their environment (Allport, 1937; Larsen and Buss, 2005). In the context of parenting a child with chronic pain, numerous parental personality factors and traits warrant attention, including trait anxiety, pain-related catastrophizing, trait mindfulness, perfectionism, and empathy.

Individuals with high levels of trait anxiety are known to selectively attend to threat stimuli (MacLeod and Mathews, 1988). When caring for a child with chronic pain, high trait-anxiety parents are more likely to engage in monitoring and solicitous behaviours (Link and Fortier, 2016). Similarly, parental pain-related catastrophizing has been associated with more parental solicitous, protective, and monitoring behaviours (Frerker et al., 2016; Jaaniste et al., 2016; Langer et al., 2017). Higher levels of parental catastrophizing at the commencement of paediatric pain programmes have been associated with less change in parental solicitous behaviour during treatment (Frerker et al., 2016). Catastrophizing commonly incorporates a component of rumination, namely focused attention on the source of one's distress and its possible causes and consequences, but not a constructive consideration of possible solutions

Table 4.1 Parent behaviours and attitudes in response to their child's chronic pain

Parental behaviour or attitude	Description	Overall impact on the child's functional outcomes	Key references
Behaviours			
Validation	Communicating that a person's thoughts, feelings and pain are understandable and legitimate	Helpful	Edmond and Keefe, 2015 (review paper)
Distraction	Focussing one's own and/or child's attention away from the pain and onto other stimuli	Helpful (usually)	Walker et al., 2006
Modelling	Intentional or unintentional demonstrations of behavioural responses; observational learning	Either	Stone and Walker, 2017
Solicitousness	Unintentional encouragement or reinforcement of the child's pain or pain behaviour	Unhelpful	Evans et al., 2016
Protective	Giving the child special attention and limiting normal activities and responsibilities	Unhelpful	DuPen et al., 2016
Monitoring/ Attending	Focussing attention on the child's pain and pain behaviours	Unhelpful	Walker et al., 2006
Minimization	Discounting the child's pain and criticizing as excessive	Unhelpful	Claar et al., 2008
Attitudes			
Acceptance of pain	The process of allowing room for unpleasant thoughts and feelings rather than trying to suppress them.	Helpful	Simons et al., 2015
Psychological flexibility	The capacity to persist with or change behaviour, depending on one's values and the current situation	Helpful	Wallace et al., 2016
Mindfulness	A mental state of awareness and openness to present experiences and situations.	Helpful	Coatsworth et al., 2015 (not paediatric chronic pain sample)
Fear and avoidance	Parental fear of the child's pain and pain behaviours resulting in an avoidance of situations that might provoke pain.	Unhelpful	Simons et al., 2015
Pain catastrophizing	An exaggerated negative orientation by parents to their child's actual or anticipated pain experiences.	Unhelpful	Langer et al., 2017

(Nolen-Hoeksema et al., 2002). Consequently, catastrophizing may be associated with impaired problem-solving.

Trait mindfulness refers to a proclivity to adopt a mental state of awareness for experiences occurring in the present (Baer et al., 2006). Although mindfulness has been regarded as a relatively stable cognitive style, the inclusion of mindful parenting components into empirically validated parenting programmes has been found to enhance their effects (Coatsworth et al., 2010). Within the context of paediatric pain, parenting interventions that have incorporated mindfulness components, within an Acceptance and Commitment Therapy (ACT) framework, have found promising results (Wallace et al., 2016).

Although perfectionism in adults is associated with more emotional difficulties in children (Appleton et al., 2010; Hamilton and Schweitzer, 2000), parental perfectionism has only recently been identified as a factor associated with the paediatric chronic pain experience. Randall and colleagues (2017) found that parents of children with chronic pain, who perceived pressures from other people to be perfect, or who expected others to be perfect, had children who reported greater pain-related distress and dysfunction. Further research is needed to clarify the mechanisms of this association.

Empathy has been defined as a sense of knowing the personal experience of another person (Goubert et al., 2005), encapsulating a cognitive appreciation, as well as an affective and behavioural response (Goubert et al., 2009). With regard to parenting a child with chronic pain, parental empathy levels have been found to be associated with parental distress and concern for their child (Goubert et al., 2008). One may speculate that high levels of parental empathy in the context of paediatric chronic pain may impede a parent's ability to encourage activation despite pain.

Although such parental traits and personality factors are not easily modifiable, it may be useful for clinicians to be aware of these factors so that they can better understand why parents respond in particular ways. Future research may consider the potential value of tailoring parent-based pain interventions to key parental personality factors.

Parental appraisal and response to their child's pain

Cognitive appraisal is the process by which an individual interprets a situation and their own capacity to respond to it. The meaning one gives to a situation will impact how they respond emotionally and behaviourally. How a parent appraises their child's pain and pain behaviours may be shaped by their past experience, learning, or by information provided by health professionals. For example, parental perceptions of the high threat value of the pain not only influences their sensitivity in detecting their child's pain (Vervoort et al., 2012), but will likely increase parental monitoring and solicitous behaviours. Parent-focused paediatric pain interventions commonly focus on modifying parental appraisal and understanding of pain as needed, with the goal of optimizing the parental pain responses (Rook and Gauntlett-Gilbert, 2016).

How a parent appraises their child's coping ability will also influence their own behaviour. A study found that parents who reported lower confidence in their child's ability to cope with the pain used more protective, monitoring, and distracting behaviours, and took more days off work, even when controlling for the child's functioning (Jaaniste et al., 2016).

Resilience factors and parental response to pain

Parental resilience refers to the ability of parents to deliver quality parenting even in the face of adverse circumstances (Gavidia-Payne et al., 2015). In a paediatric chronic pain context, resilient parenting requires the ability to garner the necessary internal and external resources to manage their child's pain, whilst also providing broader quality parenting. Notably, though, parents not only need to have the capacity to both navigate their way to and access beneficial external resources, such as supportive friends and quality pain management treatment, but these resources need to be available to them.

It is not well understood what factors are associated with resilient parenting in the context of children's pain. However, parental factors associated with resilient child outcomes in the chronic pain context include parental modelling of active coping, parent promotion of behavioural activation, parental acceptance of pain, parental psychological flexibility, and positive familial interactions (Cousins et al., 2015). Whilst parental interventions within paediatric pain programmes commonly advise parents of the value of such parental responses, changing long-standing behaviours is difficult. Parents who report better psychological and physical well-being, better social support, and positive marital relations, are more likely to be able to make the necessary changes to their own behaviour.

Risk factors and parental response to a child's pain

Dealing with a stressor, such as a child's chronic pain, typically requires significant parental coping resources, representing an aspect of 'work' associated with parenting. If an individual's coping resources are already compromised, they are less likely to be able to respond adaptively. Parental emotional distress can adversely influence a child's experience and response to pain (Logan and Scharff, 2005; Palermo et al., 2014). Parents who face competing life stressors may struggle to be responsive to pain interventions which often require them to modify the way they appraise and respond to their child's pain behaviours (Rook and Gauntlett-Gilbert, 2016). Depending on the severity of parental psychological difficulties, preliminary or concurrent parent-focused interventions may be required to facilitate parental engagement in their child's pain interventions. Failing that, it may be necessary to involve an alternative family member in the child's pain intervention (Rook and Gauntlett-Gilbert, 2016).

Parental gender and cultural factors on parental response to a child's pain

There is a small body of literature outlining gender similarities and differences in how parents respond to a child's pain and how parents respond to paediatric pain interventions. Mothers have been found to engage in more catastrophizing about their child's pain (Hechler et al., 2011). Maternal, but not paternal, catastrophizing about a child's pain has been associated with the child's pain intensity (Hechler et al., 2011). Higher levels of parental catastrophizing at treatment commencement have been found to be associated with less reduction in parental solicitous behaviour (Frerker et al., 2016). Another study found mothers to respond to a pain programme with greater reductions in protective responses than fathers (Sieberg et al., 2017).

Although data are extremely limited, racial and cultural differences may also contribute to differences in how parents respond to their child's chronic pain (El-Behadli et al., 2017). For example, in the context of responding to a child with chronic pain, black parents and Hispanic parents have been found more likely to engage in protective and monitoring behaviours, relative to white parents (El-Behadli et al., 2017). Hispanic parents also engaged in more minimizing behaviours compared with white parents.

Clinical applications

This chapter has highlighted that parenting in the context of pain has an extensive impact on parental life, and that parental functioning can subsequently influence child functioning and vice versa. How this translates to best clinical practice warrants further research. Whilst parents are now commonly included in paediatric chronic pain treatment, parental involvement is varied, ranging from attendance at a single session to complete involvement (Coakley and Wihak, 2017). Moreover, although parental emotional functioning is well recognized to influence a child's pain-related functioning (Palermo et al., 2014), there is little evidence-based guidance for how parental distress should be managed (Palermo and Eccleston, 2009).

Whilst there is a clear argument for including parents in paediatric pain interventions, it is unclear how best to involve parents and how involvement fits within the developmental context of paediatric pain. For example, there is limited research to provide guidance regarding how the parental role should differ for pain interventions with a 5-year-old, relative to a 15-year-old. What accommodations should be made for the burgeoning autonomy of the adolescent? Further questions include whether parents should be considered as co-therapists or co-patients and how co-morbid parental problems that impact on child pain and functioning are addressed and by whom. Moreover, are improvements in parental well-being a treatment goal or should parental functioning be targeted with the aim of improving child outcomes?

Evidence of treatment effectiveness of parental-focused interventions is limited, with a Cochrane review identifying no evidence for the efficacy of psychological interventions with regard to altering parental outcomes in the specific context of paediatric chronic pain (Eccleston et al., 2015). However, use of parental problem-solving therapy in paediatric chronic pain is promising: a recent randomized controlled trial showed that this therapy used to treat paediatric chronic pain was associated with significantly reduced levels of parental catastrophizing and improved levels of parental physical functioning post intervention with some maintained improvements at follow up (Palermo et al., 2016). A family-based cognitive behavioural intervention resulted in clinically meaningful reduction in parent monitoring and protective behaviours (Noel et al., 2016). An alternative treatment which commonly includes a parental focus in paediatric chronic pain is that of ACT, focusing on supporting parents to be psychologically flexible in relation to their child's pain. However, results for parental outcomes in ACT studies are limited due to small sample sizes (e.g. Wallace et al., 2016).

Future research directions

There are numerous important future research directions that could be explored in subsequent work to elucidate knowledge concerning parenting in the context of chronic pain. First, it is important to redress the maternal centric focus of existing work by ensuring that fathers are properly represented in studies to examine parenting and to enable the comparison of maternal and paternal impact and functioning. Arguably, it is also important to extend study to examine the experiences of grandparents, particularly as grandparents are increasing undertaking a greater number of caregiving roles for youth.

Second, research needs to adopt a longitudinal approach to studying parents and youth over time. To date, most studies have adopted a cross-sectional perspective to examining parental impact of paediatric pain or parental pain. Following parents and families over multiple time points is especially important in a paediatric setting where changes in pain-related functioning and impact can seem magnified due to rapid changes in the development of youth.

Third, considering the complex association between parental emotional factors and paediatric pain, more research is needed to identify how parent factors should most effectively be addressed. Research into resilient parenting is also warranted.

Furthermore, further research into dyadic parent–child interactions is warranted. Utilizing models such as APIM (Cook and Kenny, 2005) will enable researchers to focus on examining the effects of one member of the dyad on the other. Such research may use smartphones or equivalent technology to capture dyadic pain interactions in real time (Connelly et al., 2017). This focus on interdependence is critical in the field of paediatric pain where a bi-directional relationship exists between parental and child functioning.

Conclusions

This chapter has demonstrated the wide-reaching impact of paediatric chronic pain on parents, particularly mothers, demonstrating impacted parental physical, psychological and social functioning. Discussion has highlighted the importance of addressing parental outcomes related to well-being, both in the context of parenting a young person with chronic pain but also for parents who themselves experience chronic pain. These findings have implications for the involvement of parents in chronic pain treatment and questions have been raised about how treatment might usefully address parental needs in addition to treating youth with chronic pain.

Parental responses to managing chronic pain in a child have been reviewed in this chapter, highlighting the implications of particular 'helpful' and 'unhelpful' responses for both parental and child outcomes. Subsequent discussion has highlighted the importance of considering parental personality in treatment settings and how treatment can usefully focus on changing how parents respond to their child's pain and to reduce parental risk factors in the context of parenting a child or adolescent with chronic pain. Studies focusing on addressing parental resilience in the face of pain, parental empathy, and dyadic responses may be particularly fruitful as will those which follow youth and parents over multiple time points.

References

Allport, G. (1937) *Personality: A Psychological Interpretation.* New York: Holt.

Appleton, P. R., Hall, H. K., and Hill, A. P. (2010) Family patterns of perfectionism: An examination of elite junior athletes and their parents. *Journal of Psychology of Sport and Exercise*, **11**, 363–71.

Armstrong, M. I., Birnie-Lefcovitch, S., and Ungar, M. T. (2005) Pathways between social support, family well-being, quality of parenting, and child resilience: What we know. *Journal of Child and Family Studies*, **14**, 269–81.

Baer, R. A. Smith, G. T., Hopkins, J., Krieremeyer, J., and Leslie, T. (2006) Using self-report assessment methods to explore facets of mindfulness. *Assessment*, **13**, 27–45.

Birnie, K. A, Chambers, C. T., Chorney, J. Fernandez, C. V., and McGrath, P. J. (2016) Dyadic analysis of child and parent trait and state pain catastrophizing in the process of children's pain communication. *Pain*, **157**, 938–48.

Birnie, K A., Chorney, J., El-Hawary, R., and PORSCHE study group (2017) Child and parent pain catastrophizing and pain from presurgery to 6 weeks postsurgery. *Pain*, **158**, 1886–1892.

Bornstein, M. H. (2006) Parenting: science and practice. in Renninger, K.A., Sigel, I. E., Damon, W. and Lerner, R. M. et al. (eds) *Handbook of Child Psychology: Child Psychology in Practice*. New Jersey: John Wiley & Sons, 893–949.

Campo, J. V., Bridge, J., Lucas, A., Savorelli, S., Walker, L., Di Lorenzo, C., et al. (2007) Physical and emotional health of mothers of youth with functional abdominal pain. *Archives of Pediatrics & Adolescent Medicine*, **161**, 131–7.

Claar, R. L., Simons, L. E., and Logan, D. E. (2008) Parental response to children's pain: The moderating impact of children's emotional distress on symptoms and disability. *Pain*, **138**, 172–9.

Coakley, R., and Wihak, T. (2017) Evidence-based psychological interventions for the management of pediatric chronic pain: New directions in research and clinical practice. *Children*, **4**, 9.

Coatsworth, J. D., Duncan, L. G., Greenberg, M. T., and Nix, R. L. (2010) Changing parent's mindfulness, child management skills and relationship quality with their youth: Results from a randomized pilot intervention trial. *Journal of Child and Family Studies*, **19**, 203–17.

Coatsworth, J. D., Duncan, L. G., Nix, R. L., Greenberg, M. T., Gayles J. G., Bamberger, K. T., et al. (2015) Integrating mindfulness with parent training: Effects of the mindfulness-enhanced strengthening families program. *Developmental Psychology*, **51**, 26–35.

Cohen, L. L., Vowles, K. E., and Eccleston, C. (2010) Parenting an adolescent with chronic pain: An investigation of how a taxonomy of adolescent functioning relates to parent distress. *Journal of Pediatric Psychology*, **35**, 748–57.

Connelly, M., Bromberg, M. H., Anthony, K. K., Gil, K. M., and Schanberg, L. E. (2017) Use of smartphones to prospectively evaluate predictors and outcomes of caregiver responses to pain in youth with chronic disease. *Pain*, **158**, 629–36.

Cook, W. L., and Kenny, D. A. (2005) The Actor–Partner Interdependence Model: A model of bidirectional effects in developmental studies. *International Journal of Behavioral Development,* **29**, 101–9.

Cousins, L. A., Kalapurakkel, S., Cohen, L. L., and Simons, L. E. (2015) Topical review: Resilience resources and mechanisms in pediatric chronic pain. *Journal of Pediatric Psychology,* **40**, 840–5.

Craig, K. D. (2009) The social communication model of pain. *Pain,* **50**, 22–32.

Craig, K. D. (2015) Social communication model of pain. *Pain,* **156**, 1198–99.

Crawford, J. (2011) Bringing it together: Assessing parenting capacity in the child protection context. *Social Work Now,* **47**, 15–26.

Crittenden, P. M. (1999) Danger and development : The organization of self-protective strategies. In: Vondra, J. I., and Barnett, D. (eds) *Atypical Attachment in Infancy and Early Childhood among Children at Developmental Risk. Monographs of the Society for Research on Child Development.* Malden: MA: Wiley-Blackwell, 145–71.

Darlington, A. S. E., Verhulst, F. C., Ormel, J., Passchier, J., and Hunfeld, J. A. M. (2011) The influence of maternal vulnerability and parenting stress on chronic pain in adolescents in a general population sample: The TRAILS study. *European Journal of Pain,* **16**, 150–9.

Donnelly, T. J., and Jaaniste, T. (2016) Attachment and chronic pain in children and adolescents. *Children,* **3**, 21.

DuPen, M., van Tilburg, M., Langer, S., Murphy, T., Romano, J., and Levy, R. (2016) Parental protectiveness mediates the association between parent-perceived child self-efficacy and health outcomes in pediatric functional abdominal pain disorder. *Children,* **3**, 15.

Eccleston, C., Crombez, G., Scotford, A., Clinch, J., and Connell, H. (2004) Adolescent chronic pain: Patterns and predictors of emotional distress in adolescents with chronic pain and their parents. *Pain,* **108**, 221–9.

Eccleston, C., Wastell, S., Crombez, G., and Jordan, A. (2008) Adolescent social development and chronic pain. *European Journal of Pain,* **12**, 765–74.

Eccleston, C., Fisher, E., Law, E., Bartlett, J., and Palermo, T. M. (2015) Psychological interventions for parents of children and adolescents with chronic illness (Review). *Cochrane Database of Systematic Reviews,* CD009660.

Edmond, S. N., and Keefe, F. J. (2015) Validating pain communication. *Pain,* **156**, 215–19.

El-Behadli, A. F., Gansert, P., and Logan, D. E. (2017) Racial differences in parental responses to children's chronic pain. *The Clinical Journal of Pain,* **33**, 503–8.

Evans, S., Payne, L., Seidman, L., Lung, K., Zeltzer, L., and Tsao, J. (2016) Maternal anxiety and children's laboratory pain: The mediating role of solicitousness. *Children,* **3**, 10.

Evans, S., Shipton, E. A., and Keenan, T. R. (2005) Psychosocial functioning of mothers with chronic pain: A comparison to pain-free controls. *European Journal of Pain,* **9**, 683–90.

Evans, S., and de Souza, L. (2008) Dealing with chronic pain: Giving voice to the experiences ofmothers with chronic pain and their children. *Qualitative Health Research,* **18**, 489–500.

Fales, J. L., Essner, B. S., Harris, M. A., and Palermo, T. M. (2014) When helping hurts: Miscarried helping in families of youth with chronic pain. *Journal of Pediatric Psychology,* **39**, 427–37.

Fayaz, A., Croft, P., Langford, R. M., Donaldson, L. J., and Jones, G. T. (2016) Prevalence of chronic pain in the UK: A systematic review and meta-analysis of population studies. *BMJ Open,* **6**, e010364.

Frerker, M., Hechler, T., Schmidt, P., and Zernikow, B. (2016) Pain-related parental behavior: Maternal and paternal responses to chronic pain of their child and modifications following inpatient interdisciplinary pain treatment. *Schmerz*, **30**, 241–7.

Gavidia-Payne, S., Denny, B., Davis, K., Francis, A., and Jackson, M. (2015) Parental resilience: A neglected construct in resilience research. *Clinical Psychologist*, **19**, 111–21.

Goubert, L. Craig, K. D., Vervoort, T., Morley, S., Sullivan, M. J., Williams A. C. de C., et al. (2005) Facing others in pain: The effects of empathy. *Pain*, **118**, 285–8.

Goubert, L., Vervoort, T., Sullivan, M. J. L., Verhoeven, K., and Crombez, G. (2008) Parental emotional responses to their child's pain: The role of dispositional empathy and catastrophizing about their child's pain. *The Journal of Pain*, **9**, 272–9.

Goubert, L., Craig, K. D., and Buysse, A. (2009) Perceiving others in pain: Experimental and clinical evidence on the role of empathy. In: Decety, J., and Ickes, W. (eds) *The Social Neuroscience of Empathy*. Massachusets: MIT Press, 53–165.

Groenewald, C. B., Essner, B. S., Wright, D., Fesinmeyer, M. D., and Palermo, T. M. (2014) The economic costs of chronic pain among a cohort of treatment seeking adolescents in the United States. *The Journal of Pain*, **15**, 925–33.

Groenewald, C. B., and Palermo, T. M. (2015) The price of pain : The economics of chronic adolescent pain. *Pain Management*, **5**, 61–4.

Hamilton, C. E. (2000) Continuity and discontinuity of attachment from infancy through adolescence. *Child Development*, **71**, 690–4.

Hamilton, T. K., and Schweitzer, R. D. (2000) The cost of being perfect: Perfectionism and suicide ideation in university students. *Australian & New Zealand Journal of Psychiatry*, **34**, 829–35.

Hechler, T., Vervoort. T., Hamann, M., Tietze, A. L., Vocks, S., Goubert, L., et al. (2011) Parental catastrophizing about their child's chronic pain: Are mothers and fathers different? *European Journal of Pain*, **15**, 515.e1–9.

Ho, I. K., Goldschneider, K. R., Kashikar-Zuck, S., Kotagal, U., Tessman, C., and Jones, B. (2008) Healthcare utilization and indirect burden among families of pediatric patients with chronic pain. *Journal of Musculoskeletal Pain*, **16**, 155–64.

Hunfeld, J. A., Perquin, C. W., Duivenvoorden, H. J., Hazebroek-Kampschreur, A. A., Passchier, J., van Suijlekom-Smit, L. W., and van der Wouden, J. C. (2001) Chronic pain and its impact on quality of life in adolescents and their families. *Journal of Pediatric Psychology*, **26**, 145–53.

Jaaniste, T. Jia, N., Lang, T., Goodison-Farnsworth, E. M., McCormick, M., and Anderson, D. (2016) The relationship between parental attitudes and behaviours in the context of paediatric chronic pain. *Child Care Health and Development*, **42**, 433–8.

Jordan, A., Crabtree, A., and Eccleston, C. (2016) You have to be a jack of all trades': Fathers parenting their adolescent with chronic pain. *Journal of Health Psychology*, **21**, 2466–76.

Jordan, A. L., Eccleston, C., and Osborn, M. (2007) Being a parent of the adolescent with complex chronic pain: An interpretative phenomenological analysis. *European Journal of Pain*, **11**, 49–56.

Langer, S. L., Romano, J., Brown, J. D., Nielson, H., Ou, B., Rauch, C., et al. (2017) Sequential analysis of child pain behavior and maternal responses. *Pain*, **158**, 1678–86.

Larsen, R., and Buss, D. (2005) *Personality Psychology: Domains of Knowledge About Human Nature*. 2nd edn. McGraw Hill: New York.

Lewandowski, A. S., Palermo, T. M., Stinson, J., Handley, S., and Chambers, C. T. (2010) Systematic review of family functioning in families of children and adolescents with chronic pain. *The Journal of Pain*, 11, 1027–38.

Link, C.J., and Fortier, M.A. (2016) The relationship between parent trait anxiety and parent-reported pain, solicitous behaviors, and quality of life impairment in children with cancer. *Journal of Pediatric Hematology/Oncology*, 38, 58–62.

Logan, D. E., and Scharff, L. (2005) Relations between family and parent characteristics and functional disabilities in children with recurrent pain syndromes: An investigation of moderating effects on the pathways from pain to disability. *Journal of Pediatric Psychology*, 30, 698–707.

Maciver, D., Jones, D., and Nicol, M. (2010) Parents' experiences of caring for a child with chronic pain. *Qualitative Health Research*, 20, 1272–82.

MacLeod, C., and Mathews, A. (1988) Anxiety and the allocation of attention to threat. *Human Experimental Psychology*, 40, 653–70.

Mahrer, N. E., Gold, J. I., Luu, M., and Herman, P. M. (2018) A cost-analysis of an interdisciplinary pediatric chronic pain clinic. *Journal of Pain*, 19, 158–65.

Malekpour, M. (2007) Effects of attachment on early and later development. *The British Journal of Development Disabilities*, 53, 81–95.

Mano, K. E. J., Khan, K. A., Ladwig, R. J., and Weisman, S. J. (2011) The impact of pediatric chronic pain on parents' health-related quality of life and family functioning: Reliability and validity of the PedsQL 4.0 Family Impact Module. *Journal of Pediatric Psychology*, 36, 517–27.

McKillop, H., and Banez, G. (2016) A broad consideration of risk factors in pediatric chronic pain: Where to go from here? *Children*, 3, 38.

Meltzer, L. J., and Moore, M. (2008) Sleep disruptions in parents of children and adolescents with chronic illnesses: Prevalence, causes, and consequences. *Journal of Pediatric Psychology*, 33, 279–91.

Minuchin, S., Baker, L., Rosmna, B. L., Liebman, R., Milman, L., and Todd, T. C. (1975) A conceptual model of psychosomatic illness in children. Family organization and family therapy. *Archives of General Psychiatry*, 32, 1031–8.

Neville, A., Soltani, S., Pavlova, M., and Noel, M. (2018) Unravelling the relationship between parent and child PTSD and pediatric chronic pain: The mediating role of pain catastrophizing. *Journal of Pain*, 19, 196–206.

Noel, M., Alberts, N., Langer, S. L., Levy, R. L., Walker, L. S., and Palermo, T. M. (2016) The sensitivity to change and responsiveness of the Adult Responses to Children's Symptoms in children and adolescents with chronic pain. *Journal of Pediatric Psychology*, 41, 350–62.

Nolen-Hoeksema, S., Wisco, B. E., and Lyubomirsky, S. (2002) Rethinking rumination. *Perspectives on Psychological Science*, 5, 400–24.

Palermo, T. M., Law, E. F., Essner, B. M, Jessen-Fiddick, T., and Eccleston, C. (2014) Adaptation of problem-solving skills training (PSST) for parent caregivers of youth with chronic pain. *Clinical Practice in Pediatric Psychology*, 2, 212–23.

Palermo, T. M., Law, E. F., Bromberg, M. H., Fales, J., Eccleston, C., and Wilson, A.C. (2016) Problem-solving skills training for parents of children with chronic pain. *Pain*, 157, 1213–23.

Palermo, T. M., and Eccleston, C. (2009) Parents of children and adolescents with chronic pain. *Pain*, 146, 15–17.

Palermo, T. M., Valrie, C. R., and Karlson, C. W. (2014) Family and parent influences on pediatric chronic pain A developmental perspective. *American Psychologist*, 69, 142–52.

Randall, E. T., Smith, K. R., Kronman, C. A., Conroy, C., Smith, A. M., and Simons, L. E. (2017) Feeling the pressure to be perfect: Impact on pain-related distress and dysfunction in youth with chronic pain. *The Journal of Pain*, **19**, 418–29.

Rook, S., and Gauntlett-Gilbert, J. (2016) Parent involvement in pediatric pain interventions. *Pediatric Pain Letter*, **18**, 9–13.

Sieberg, C. B., Smith, A., White, M., Manganella, J., Sethna, N. and Logan, E. E. (2017) Changes in maternal and paternal pain-related attitudes, behaviors, and perceptions across pediatric pain rehabilitation treatment: A multilevel modeling approach. *Journal of Pediatric Psychology*, **43**, 52–64.

Simons, L. E., Smith, A., Kaczynski, K., and Basch, M. (2015) Living in fear of your child's pain: The Parent Fear of Pain Questionnaire. *Pain*, **156**, 694–702.

Sleed, M., Eccleston, C., Beecham, J., Knapp, M., and Jordan. A. (2005) The economic impact of chronic pain in adolescence: Methodological considerations and a preliminary costs-of-illness study. *Pain*, **119**, 183–90.

Stone, A. L., Bruehl, S., Smith, C. A., Garber, J., and Walker, L. (2018) Social learning pathways in the relation between parental chronic pain and daily pain severity and functional impairment in adolescents with functional abdominal pain. *Pain*, **159**, 298–305.

Stone, A. L., and Walker, L. S. (2017) Adolescents' observations of parent pain behaviors: Preliminary measure validation and test of social learning theory in pediatric chronic pain. *Journal of Pediatric Psychology*, **42**, 65–74.

Timko, C., Stovel, K. W., and Moos, R. H. (1992) Functioning among mothers and fathers of children with juvenile rheumatic disease: A longitudinal study. *Journal of Pediatric Psychology*, **17**, 705–24.

Umberger, W. A., and Risko, J. (2016) 'It didn't kill me. It just made me stronger and wiser': Silver linings for children and adolescents of parents with chronic pain. *Archives of Psychiatric Nursing*, **30**, 138–43.

Vervoort, T., Caes, L., Trost, Z., Notebaert, L., and Goubert, L. (2012) Parental attention to their child's pain is modulated by threat-value of pain. *Health Psychology*, **31**, 623–31.

Walker, L. S., Williams, S. E., Smith, C. A., Garber, J., Van Slyke, D. A., and Lipani, T. A. (2006) Parent attention versus distraction: Impact on symptom complaints by children with and without chronic functional abdominal pain. *Pain*, **122**, 43–52.

Wallace, D. P., Woodford, B., and Connelly, M. (2016) Promoting psychological flexibility in parents of adolescents with chronic pain : Pilot study of an 8-week group intervention. *Clinical Practice in Pediatric Psychology*, **4**, 405–16.

Wilson, A. C., and Fales, J. (2016) Parenting in the context of chronic pain: A controlled study of parents with chronic pain. *Clinical Journal of Pain*, **31**, 689–98.

Chapter 5

The impact of chronic pain on school functioning in young people

Line Caes and Deirdre Logan

The importance of the school environment in childhood development

School plays a central role in young people's lives. It is not only the place where young people spend the majority of their waking hours, it also makes a crucial contribution to development. Beyond teaching key skills and knowledge, the school environment stimulates the development of independence, identity, cognitive-emotional functioning, and social skills (Sato et al., 2007). Indeed, while the role of the school environment in social learning is often overlooked, in school young people learn how to build relationships with peers and adults alike. Schools are therefore a central place for young people to form and maintain friendships, and develop social competency and a sense of self, which are all fundamental to long-term functioning and well-being throughout adulthood (Shui, 2001).

Consequently, extensive absence from school is problematic. School absence not only negatively influences academic performance but also hinders social, emotional, and cognitive development. Indeed, chronic absenteeism, sometimes referred to as school refusal or avoidance if absences are unexcused, is a risk factor for a myriad of mental and physical health problems such as suicide, unsafe sexual behaviour, violence, substance abuse, economic deprivation, school dropout, psychiatric disorders, and marital problems (Kearney, 2008). Sometimes school absences are 'excused' due to medical reasons. The distinction between missing school for medical or behavioural reasons is not always clear-cut, however. For young people with chronic medical conditions, many behavioural factors beyond their symptoms influence their ability or inability to attend school.

To fully understand the impact of school absenteeism, it is important to recognize that school absenteeism is a complex phenomenon, influenced by many temporal, cognitive, and developmental factors (Kearney, 2008; Sato et al., 2007). For instance, while irrational school-related fears influence school absenteeism to a large extent, the content of the fears tends to look different across developmental stages: while separation fear from parents is highly prevalent in young children, older children report more social-evaluative fears (fear of evaluations by teachers and other young people; King, et al., 1995).

The school environment, in particular the young person's relation with their teacher(s), can influence absenteeism. A positive teacher–student relationship has been described as 'the degree to which students feel respected, supported, and valued by their teachers' (Suldo et al., 2009, p. 68). Indeed, teaching styles which support the development of and need for autonomy and competence can have far-reaching effects on young people's academic and social-emotional functioning. A supportive relationship with a teacher, especially one providing emotional and informational support, can not only improve school functioning, performance, dropout, and satisfaction, but also has the potential to reduce the negative impact of stress on school functioning (Suldo et al., 2009; Vervoort et al., 2014).

The prevalence of young people with extra needs, due to health conditions, disabilities, or developmental delays, attending mainstream schools has risen substantially in recent years (Magalnick and Mazyck, 2008; Shiu, 2001). Advancements in medical treatments and technology have indeed allowed more young people with a chronic illness to remain in schools and thereby form an integral part of the school community (Shiu, 2001). However, meeting the individual needs of young people with chronic illnesses in schools is an increasing challenge. This chapter will focus on young people experiencing chronic pain. Evidence shows that chronic pain in young people influences school participation, attendance, academic achievement, peer relationships, and perceived competence in academic and social domains (Dick and Riddell, 2010; Gorodzinsky et al., 2011; Logan, Simons et al., 2008). An overview and critical discussion will be presented on how a young person's school functioning can be negatively affected by chronic pain experiences. The chapter will end with the proposal of a comprehensive model to foster our understanding of the complex bi-directional associations between chronic pain experiences and school functioning and associated challenges for future research.

How chronic pain impacts school engagement and functioning

The experience of pain, especially chronic pain, has the potential to impose a significant burden on young people. Chronic pain can interfere with all aspects of daily functioning, characterized by impaired sleep patterns, and diminished school, physical, emotional, and social functioning (Connell, 2004; Eccleston et al., Konijnenberg et al., 2005; Logan and Scharff, 2005; Logan et al., 2008; Long et al., 2008). In the first part of this chapter, a detailed overview will be provided on the impact of the chronic pain experience on school attendance and participation, learning and academic performance, and school-based social skills.

School attendance

The most commonly evaluated impact of chronic pain on school functioning is school attendance (Logan and Simons, 2010), with evidence indicating elevated school absences in young people with chronic pain. Across various pain locations, e.g. head, abdominal, musculoskeletal, averages of missing 3 days of school each month are reported (Konijnenberg et al., 2005). A Finnish study comparing school absenteeism in young people reporting chronic musculoskeletal to pain-free children found that twice as many young people with pain reported being absent from school in the past 3 months (25.5% school absences in young people with chronic pain compared to 11.6% absences reported by pain-free young people; Mikkelsson et al., 1997). Given the strong role school plays in a young person's development, these school absences can have far-reaching consequences for cognitive, social, and emotional development. Indeed, a longitudinal study revealed positive associations between greater school absences in young people with chronic pain and increased functional disability over time (Walker et al., 2002).

Despite the frequent reliance on school absenteeism as an outcome for school functioning, a recent systematic review on measures to assess school functioning amongst young people with chronic pain highlighted several limitations with both the focus on, and assessment of, school attendance (Gorodzinsky et al., 2011). With respect to school attendance the most commonly used metric is being absent for a full day. However, despite the simplicity of this metric, most studies do not provide adequate details on their definition of school absence and a large variety of operationalizations are observed: reasons of absence are often not requested and/or reported, the timeframe to report varies from 1 month to 1 year, and different agents of report are used (e.g. most studies rely on self-report or parent report, with a handful of studies using multiple reporting agents; Gorodzinsky et al., 2011). In addition, it is common for young people with chronic pain to arrive late at school or leave school early (Logan et al., 2008); these partial-day absences are often missed through traditional means of measuring school attendance.

Beyond these methodological issues it is also important to acknowledge that school functioning encompasses more than just attending school. A thorough understanding and assessment of how chronic pain impacts school functioning should include the impact on academic performance, academic competence, participation in school activities, and social functioning in the school setting (Gorodzinsky et al., 2011). Related to this broader perspective on school functioning, evidence is accumulating to suggest that school absence in young people with chronic pain is not merely related to pain intensity or duration but also that psychosocial and other behavioural factors are often involved (Logan et al., 2008). Indeed, the link between chronic pain and sleep deprivation, dysfunctional family relations, as well as mental health difficulties (e.g. increased levels of anxiety and depression) could contribute to the impact of pain-related school functioning (Gorodzinsky et al., 2011).

The impact of mental health difficulties experienced by young people with chronic pain on school attendance and functioning in particular is gaining research attention. For instance, depressive symptoms were found to significantly influence various indicators of school functioning in young people with chronic pain, including school absence (Logan et al., 2009). Furthermore, even when controlling for pain intensity, Khan and colleagues (2015) found a direct influence of anxiety on poor school functioning, including attendance, school avoidance behaviours, and academic difficulties. Social influences are also important to consider. For example, parental responses to pain symptoms have been shown to influence school functioning among youth with chronic pain, with parents' negative thinking about pain playing a mechanistic role (Logan et al., 2012). Beyond the impact of parents, teacher support has been found to buffer the negative impact of pain experiences on school functioning (Vervoort et al., 2014). The role of teacher support will be discussed in more depth later within this chapter.

Taken together, these findings suggest that beyond pain, psychosocial factors may substantially contribute to problematic school functioning in young people with chronic pain. In the next two sections, we go beyond school attendance and provide an overview of how chronic pain in young people, and associated psychosocial factors, influence broader aspects of school functioning. We first highlight the impact on learning and academic performance, followed by the impact on social development.

Academic performance

Findings using standardized assessments, such as the Quality of Life Inventory (PedsQL, Varni et al., 2006), Harter Self-Perception Profile for Adolescents (Harter, 1988), or standard batteries for general intelligence (IQ), have revealed poorer overall school functioning in young people with chronic pain compared to young people with less severe disease states and pain-free young people (Gorodzinsky et al., 2011). However, no differences in general cognitive competence between young people with and without chronic pain have emerged (Haverkamp et al., 2002; Ho et al., 2009). Studies examining specific domains of school functioning have yielded mixed findings. Some studies showed a decrease in perceived academic competence compared to pain-free peers (Walker et al., 1998) while others found no differences (Logan et al., 2008). Logan and colleagues (2008) did, however, show a self-reported decline in grades and in subjective perceptions of school success among young people asked to compare their functioning before and after pain onset (Logan et al., 2008). Looking at a specific aspect of academic performance, a population-based study by Kosola and colleagues (2018) revealed that primary school children (aged 8–9 years) with chronic pain showed a significant delay in their reading and numeracy skill compared to pain-free peers. A potential explanation of these differences might be the complexity of how chronic pain can impact academic performance, with potential mediating factors not being accounted for. For instance, depressive symptoms have been found to influence self-reported academic performance, self- and parent-reported pain interferences, and teachers' ratings of adjustment to school (Logan et al., 2009).

The lack of comprehensive assessments appropriate for the context of chronic pain has resulted in the use of non-standardized assessments, further increasing the difficulties of comparing findings. Using such non-standardized assessments, evidence suggests that young people with chronic pain report lower satisfaction with school (Carlsson et al., 1996) and difficulties in completing school-related sports and activities (Walters and Williamson, 2000), as well as a lower ability to maintain concentration, effort, and motivation during classes (Bonner et al., 1999). Furthermore, this reduced engagement with school-related activities was not only influenced by pain but also due to associated pain-related sleep deprivation (Bonner et al., 1999) and linked to higher levels of depressive symptoms (Walters and Williamson, 2000). Although the evidence is mixed, pain medications (e.g. opioids, tricyclic antidepressants (TCA), and anticonvulsant drugs) have also been found to contribute to worse cognitive functioning (Chapman et al., 2002; Moriarty et al., 2011). Research evaluating the impact of pain medication on cognitive functioning in paediatric populations is lacking and further exploration of the underlying mechanisms by which pain medication affects cognitive functioning is warranted. Nevertheless, these findings reveal the importance of controlling for the role of analgesic medication when investigating the associations between paediatric chronic pain and school functioning.

As the subjectivity of self-reports potentially contributes to the disparities found with academic performance, using cognitive tests to assess cognitive functioning in general could shed more light on the impact of pain on specific aspects of cognitive functioning relevant for academic performance. A 2010 critical review (Dick and Pillai Riddell, 2010) summarized the limited evidence on this topic. Preliminary evidence indicates that young people with chronic pain show specific impairments in their attention, expressed as difficulties in attending to non-pain information combined with difficulties in disengaging attention from pain (e.g. Boyer et al., 2005; Zohsel et al., 2008), and a memory bias towards pain-related information (Koutantji et al., 1999). More recently, preliminary pilot data from a small sample of female adolescents with chronic pain ($N = 13$) revealed reduced working memory capacity and selective attention, using standardized neurocognitive tests, compared to matched pain-free adolescents (Mifflin et al., 2016). Importantly, Hocking and colleagues (2010) identified that selective attention plays an important role in explaining coping mechanisms adopted by youth with recurrent functional abdominal pain, which in turn was also related to lower levels of anxiety. Further replication of these findings in larger and more diverse samples of young people with chronic pain is needed to gain a comprehensive understanding of associations among cognitive functioning, chronic pain, and academic performance (Dick and Pillai Riddell, 2010). Indeed, evidence in adults with chronic pain indicates that the experience of chronic pain has the potential to impede the effectiveness of executive functioning, such as decision-making, and emotional self-regulation (Berryman et al., 2014; Moriarty et al., 2011). Given that young people with chronic pain tend to miss out on more school days compared to pain-free young people, impairments in cognitive functioning, such as executive functioning, could add an extra layer of difficulties by increased difficulty to keep up with missed academic material (Mifflin et al., 2016). Further research is also needed to investigate the reverse causal pathway: that is, the possibility that learning challenges such as executive functioning deficits might increase vulnerability for developing chronic pain conditions, possibly through heightened stress (Kosola et al., 2017).

Beyond the assessment issues with academic performance, a lifespan approach towards academic performance in youth with pain is absent from the literature. Indeed, there is a lack of longitudinal evaluations of factors influencing academic performance as well as how impaired academic performance influences career opportunities in adulthood. On the other end of the spectrum, our understanding is limited on how repeated exposure to painful experiences early in life influences academic performance. While evidence is emerging on how repeated pain experiences in neonates impacts their pain sensitivity later in childhood, there is an urgent need for long-term studies to evaluate the impact of early pain exposure on neurodevelopment and associated skills such as cognitive and academic performance (Grunau et al., 2006).

Social skills

Missing school can have wider implications beyond impairing academic performance. In particular, the school environment is a crucial place to connect with same-aged peers and experiment with building and maintaining friendships within a safe environment. However, due to frequent absences, young people with chronic pain have reduced opportunities to explore and refine these developing social skills (Merlijn et al., 2003). The development of these social skills to adaptively connect with peers is of major importance during adolescence, as this stage is characterized by a desire for more autonomy from parents and consequently more reliance on peers for support. In accordance with these assumptions, it has been found that adolescents with chronic pain perceive themselves as less socially accepted by their peers (Merlijn et al., 2003) and less developed, compared to their peers, particularly with respect to confidence in social situations, their future, independence, and identity development (Eccleston et al., 2008). Importantly, the most commonly reported perceived disparity compared to their peers was found for school progress and independence (Eccleston et al., 2008). Highlighting the complexity of these associations, recent evidence from a large community sample revealed the role of pain-related anxiety in understanding the impact of chronic pain on social development. In particular, increased levels of pain-related anxiety were found to contribute to heightened perceptions of social impairment compared to their pain-free peers but only amongst female adolescents with chronic pain (Caes et al., 2015).

Perceived social competence is vital to the development of healthy friendships. Despite the importance of friendships in young people's social development, and how adaptive school functioning can facilitate this development, our knowledge on how chronic pain experiences influence friendships is limited. A systematic review summarizing the limited evidence across chronic pain types revealed that young people with chronic pain participate in fewer peer activities, have fewer friends, and are perceived as more isolated than their pain-free peers (Forgeron et al., 2010). However, few studies have focused on the extent to which reduced school engagement contributes to these social difficulties, such as maintaining friendships, or whether continued, regular engagement with school-related activities, despite chronic pain experiences, can act as a buffer towards social impairments due to pain. Preliminary evidence suggests a link between social and school functioning, with high levels of social functioning and positive friendships acting as a potential buffer against the negative impact of a young person's chronic pain experience and school impairment (Simons et al., 2010; Walker et al., 1994).

One particular aspect of friendship quality within a school context that is receiving increased research attention in the last decade is the role of pain experiences on peer victimization. For instance, young people experiencing recurrent abdominal pain reported increased levels of peer victimization compared to pain-free young people. This increased level of peer victimization was not only directly associated with impaired social skills, academic competence, and increased usage of school medical services, but it also intensified the negative impact of pain intensity on academic competence and medical service usage (Greco et al., 2007). However, the causality of the association between chronic pain and peer victimization is unclear. Indeed, population-based studies also identified that young people who experience frequent bullying and associated school-related stress report more pain experiences (Hjern et al., 2008; Vervoort et al., 2014). Taken together, it is unclear whether stress associated with peer victimization poses a risk factor for the development of chronic pain or whether the experience of chronic pain poses a risk for becoming a target of peer victimization (Forgeron et al., 2010). Either way, findings highlight the potentially devastating impact of a negative school environment on academic performance, thereby demonstrating the importance of positive social experiences in school.

The role of teachers

Recent research has highlighted the crucial role of teachers in creating and supporting a positive school experience. Recent evidence, gathered in a large representative sample of 10,650 Flemish-speaking school children, revealed that teachers supporting young people's competence and autonomy not only has a direct positive influence on school functioning, but it can also buffer against the negative impact of pain on school functioning (Vervoort et al., 2014). In particular, students with a teacher who supported their competence and autonomy reported better academic performance, lower school-related pressure, and higher school-related satisfaction. Furthermore, such teacher support of students' competence and autonomy also reduced the impact of pain experiences on school absenteeism. However, only teacher support of students' competence was found to buffer the impact of pain experiences on bullying (Vervoort et al., 2014). Research exploring the teachers' perspective on their experience with pain in their students has further confirmed the central role teachers can play in adaptive pain management. A focus group of Norwegian secondary school teachers ($N = 22$) revealed their understanding of how biopsychosocial factors influence pain, which was reflected in the approaches the teachers engaged in to understand and reduce their students' pain (e.g. taking time to talk with them; advising relaxation; establishing a cooperative relationship between parents and all school staff; Rhode et al., 2015).

To our knowledge, only two studies asked teachers directly about the challenges they face in accommodating the needs of students with chronic pain and their needs to overcome these challenges (Logan and Curran, 2005; Tarpey et al., 2018). Despite the studies being conducted 13 years apart and the focus being on different educational systems—US middle and high school teachers (Logan and Curran, 2005) versus Irish primary school teachers (Tarpey et al., 2018)—the identified challenges and needs were consistent. The findings of both studies highlighted how teachers are aware of their central role in supporting effective pain management within the school setting, but also indicated how high classroom numbers, curriculum overload, and the need to balance the needs of all their students often stand in the way of offering this supportive environment. Furthermore, in both studies teachers revealed their lack of knowledge on paediatric pain and practical evidence-based pain management techniques as well as the absence of any official (government-supported) resources and support for pain management within the school setting. Strategies for overcoming these challenges overlapped in both studies as well and can be summarized in two themes: provision of official training and resources on pain management and establishing effective communication channels between the school staff, parents, and health-care team (Logan and Curran, 2005; Tarpey et al., 2018).

Importantly, the findings from both these studies also indicated that the presence of a medical diagnosis for the pain experiences can be a boost to the teachers' ability to provide support. Not only did a diagnosis reduce the teachers' uncertainty about the authenticity of the pain, it also acted as a catalyst to provide official support such as one-on-one access to support staff, to assist the student with their individual needs, and to reduce the burden of the teacher. Without a diagnosis, however, access to support staff was not possible (Tarpey et al., 2018). The availability of a diagnosis or other medical evidence supporting students' pain complaints has also been found to influence teachers' perceptions of pain severity and impairment as well as their behavioural responses, such as allowing relief from responsibilities and implementing accommodations (Logan et al., 2007).

Taken together, there is limited, but growing, evidence on the central role of classroom teachers and school support staff in providing young people with a supportive school environment and on the need to provide appropriate training and support to school staff. Evaluations of the implementation and effectiveness of school-based pain management programmes deserve more research attention. For instance, while therapist-administered relaxation was more effective, compared to school nurse administration, for managing migraines and tension-type headaches in young people, school nurse administration of relaxation training did lead to clinical improvements and was rated as most efficient and cost-effective for managing tension-type headaches (Larsson et al., 2005). Another example of a creative approach is the Chronic Pain 35 programme, recently implemented by Reid and colleagues (2016). Chronic Pain 35 integrates a cognitive-behavioural chronic pain self-management programme within the school curriculum for adolescents between 14 and 18 years of age across Alberta, Canada. The innovative aspect of this Chronic Pain 35 programme is that it is set up like a school course (e.g. including mandatory face-to-face group sessions, weekly homework, assignments), thereby allowing the young people attending the programme to gain school credits for their attendance and engagement in the programme. While systematic evaluation of Chronic Pain 35 is underway, preliminary feedback from the 32 young people who completed the programme is promising. The young people particularly valued obtaining academic credits, which they might otherwise be missing out on, to be able to graduate. Beyond facilitating academic achievements, the programme was positively evaluated for forging peer connections and support as well as assisting young people in advocating for themselves, which led to improved perspectives of the teachers' understanding of the young persons' pain experience (Reid et al., 2016).

Future challenges and directions: the need for a biopsychosocial approach

Chronic pain can influence many areas of school functioning, including attendance, performance, self-concept, and social relationships. It is important to assess all of these when attempting to identify the school-based needs of any individual young person with chronic pain.

There are, however, still some barriers to overcome to facilitate such an all-encompassing approach towards school functioning in young people with chronic pain within both research and clinical practice. The main barriers we have identified include the lack of standardized, reliable, and valid assessment measures of the various aspects of school functioning, prospective designs, and the absence of a guiding theoretical framework.

The variety of assessment approaches used in the existing literature, across self-report and cognitive tests, provides an opportunity to develop a battery/library of available tools to reliably assess the various aspects of school functioning that can account for the variability between school settings. Such a tool battery or library would not only avoid inducing further variability in the adopted assessment approaches within future research on school functioning but also facilitate systematic and comparable evaluation of school functioning within clinical practice. We propose a bio-psycho-social model of school functioning in young people with chronic pain (see Figure 5.1). The model is anticipated

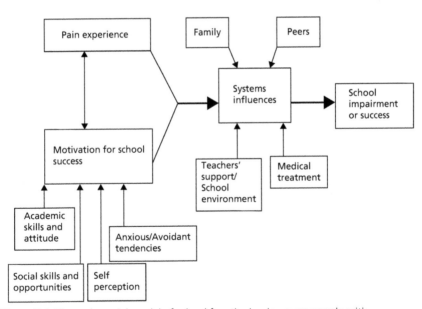

Figure 5.1 Biopsychosocial model of school functioning in young people with chronic pain

Reproduced with permission from Logan, D. E. (2013). *Exploring the role of school self-efficacy and belongingness among adolescents with chronic pain in the school setting.* Presented at the 13th meeting of the International Symposium on Pediatric Pain, Stockholm, Sweden.

to facilitate our understanding of how pain, school functioning, and the many potential modulators of the pain-school functioning pathway, on both individual and systems levels, interact to shape the school experience in the context of chronic pain. The model also acknowledges that these modulators can vary widely by individual. It is anticipated that this model will not only expand research on school functioning in young people with chronic pain, through model testing and revision, but will also inform clinical practice. For instance, understanding key contributors can elucidate important targets of intervention (e.g. for one young person the key to school success might be treating anxiety focused on the school setting, whereas for another it may be most important to help the teachers understand the pain issues and respond to the young person supportively).

Using longitudinal approaches, it will be critical to evaluate the application of this model across the various school settings: primary school; secondary school; college and university. Indeed, the majority of the evidence on how chronic pain affects school functioning is based on the experience of adolescents within secondary school settings. Limited evidence is available for young children within primary school settings (Kosola et al., 2018; Tarpey et al., 2018) as well as how chronic pain impacts students' performance within university/college settings. For instance, due to their age and lower capacity to manage their own pain, it is reasonable to assume that teachers' support might be even more important for younger children. On the other hand, given the evidence that chronic pain could impair executive functioning and the required independence with respect to time management within a university/college setting, young people with chronic pain might struggle to perform optimally at this level. Factors such as self-efficacy/self-concept, academic engagement, school attendance, and social connectedness have all been found to predict long-term academic and career achievement (Bandura et al., 2001; Bond et al., 2007; Easton and Englehard, 1982; Green et al., 2012; Harackiewicz et al., 2002; Scales et al., 2006). In light of the influence pain can have on each of these concepts, there is an urgent need for more longitudinal approaches to advance our knowledge on the potential negative impact of pain experiences on school functioning and how in turn this impaired school functioning influences future academic and career opportunities.

In conclusion, school is at the centre of young people's lives and is a vital environment for their positive development. When chronic pain disrupts a young person's life, the effects on school functioning can be extensive and wide-ranging. When working with young people with chronic pain, it is crucial to dedicate time and effort to understanding how pain intersects with and influences school functioning across these many domains. Addressing pain-related school issues and collaborating with teachers, parents, and others who can help to foster the young person's school success is of paramount importance in achieving the overall goal of restoring an adaptive path of development.

References

Bandura, A., Barbaranelli, C., Caprara, G. V., and Pastorelli C. (2001) Self-efficacy beliefs as shapers of children's aspirations and career trajectories. *Child Development*, **72**, 187–206.

Berryman, C., Stanton, T. R., Bowering, K. J., Tabor, A., McFarlane, A., and Moseley, G. L. (2014) Do people with chronic pain have impaired executive function? A meta-analytical review. *Clinical Psychology Review*, **34**, 563–79.

Bond, L., Butler, H., Thomas, L., Carlin, J., Glover, S., Bowes, G., and Patton G. (2007) Social and school connectedness in early secondary school as predictors of late teenage substance use, mental health, and academic outcomes. *Journal of Adolescent Health,* **40**, 357:e9–18.

Bonner, M. J., Gustafson, K. E., Schumacher, E., and Thompson, R. J. (1999) The impact of sickle cell disease on cognitive functioning and learning. *School Psychology Review,* **28**, 182–93.

Boyer, M. C., Compas, B. E., Stanger, C., Colletti, R. B., Konik, B. S., Morrow, S. B., and Thomsen, A. H. (2005) Attentional biases to pain and social threat in children with recurrent abdominal pain. *Journal of Pediatric Psychology,* **31**, 209–20.

Caes, L., Fisher, E., Clinch, J., Tobias, J. H., and Eccleston, C. (2015) The role of pain-related anxiety in adolescents' disability and social impairment: ALSPAC data. *European Journal of Pain,* **19**, 842–51.

Carlsson, J., Larsson, B., and Mark, A. (1996) Psychosocial functioning in schoolchildren with recurrent headaches. *Headache,* **36**, 77–82.

Chapman, S. L., Byas-Smith, M. G., and Reed, B. A. (2002) Effects of intermediate-and long-term use of opioids on cognition in patients with chronic pain. *The Clinical Journal of Pain,* **18**, S83–90.

Dick, B. D., and Riddell Pillai, R. (2010) Cognitive and school functioning in children and adolescents with chronic pain: a critical review. *Pain Research and Management,* **15**, 238–44.

Easton, J.Q., and Engelhard, Jr. G. (1982) A longitudinal record of elementary school absence and its relationship to reading achievement. *The Journal of Educational Research,* **75**, 269–74.

Eccleston, C., Crombez, G., Scotford, A., Clinch, J., and Connell. H. (2004) Adolescent chronic pain: Patterns and predictors of emotional distress in adolescents with chronic pain and their parents. *Pain,* **108**, 221–9.

Eccleston, C., Wastell, S., Crombez, G., and Jordan, A. (2008) Adolescent social development and chronic pain. *European Journal of Pain,* **12**, 765–74.

Forgeron, P. A., King, S., Stinson, J. N., McGrath, P. J., MacDonald, A. J., and Chambers, C. T. (2010) Social functioning and peer relationships in children and adolescents with chronic pain: A systematic review. *Pain Research and Management,* **15**, 27–41.

Gorodzinsky, A. Y., Hainsworth, K. R., and Weisman, S. J. (2011) School functioning and chronic pain: a review of methods and measures. *Journal of Pediatric Psychology,* **36**, 991–1002.

Greco, L. A., Freeman, K. E., and Dufton, L. (2007) Overt and relational victimization among children with frequent abdominal pain: links to social skills, academic functioning, and health service use. *Journal of Pediatric Psychology,* **32**, 319–29.

Green, J., Liem, G. A., Martin, A. J., Colmar, S., Marsh, H. W., and McInerney, D. (2012) Academic motivation, self-concept, engagement, and performance in high school: Key processes from a longitudinal perspective. *Journal of Adolescence,* **35**, 1111–22.

Grunau, R. E., Holsti, L., and Peters, J. W. (2006) Long-term consequences of pain in human neonates. *Seminars in Fetal and Neonatal Medicine,* **11**, 268–75.

Harackiewicz, J. M., Barron, K. E., Tauer, J. M., and Elliot, A. J. (2002) Predicting success in college: A longitudinal study of achievement goals and ability measures as predictors of interest and performance from freshman year through graduation. *Journal of Educational Psychology,* **94**, 562.

Harter, S. (1988) *Manual for the Self-Perception Profile for Adolescents*. Denver: University of Denver.

Haverkamp, F., Hönscheid, A., and Müller-Sinik, K. (2002) Cognitive development in children with migraine and their healthy unaffected siblings. *Headache*, **42**, 776–9.

Hjern, A., Alfven, G., and Östberg, V. (2008) School stressors, psychological complaints and psychosomatic pain. *Acta Paediatrica*, **97**, 112–17.

Ho, G. H. Y., Bennett, S. M., Cox, D., and Poole, G. (2009) Brief report: Cognitive functioning and academic achievement in children and adolescents with chronic pain. *Journal of Pediatric Psychology*, **34**, 311–316.

Hocking, M. C., Barnes, M., Shaw, C., Lochman, J. E., Madan-Swain, A., and Saeed, S. (2010) Executive function and attention regulation as predictors of coping success in youth with functional abdominal pain. *Journal of Pediatric Psychology*, **36**, 64–73.

Kearney, C. A. (2008) School absenteeism and school refusal behavior in youth: A contemporary review. *Clinical Psychology Review*, **28**, 451–71.

Khan, K. A., Tran, S. T., Mano, K. E. J., Simpson, P. M., Cao, Y., and Hainsworth, K. R. (2015) Predicting multiple facets of school functioning in pediatric chronic pain: Examining the direct impact of anxiety. *The Clinical Journal of Pain*, **31**, 867–75.

King, N. J., Ollendick, T. H., and Tonge, B. J. (1995) *School Refusal: Assessment and Treatment*. Boston: Allyn and Bacon.

Konijnenberg, A. Y., Uieterwaal, C. S. P. M., Kimpen, J. L. L., van der Hoeven, J., Buitetlaar, J. K., and de Graeff-Meeder, E. R. (2005) Children with unexplained chronic pain: substantial impairment in everyday life. *Archives of Diseases in Childhood*, **90**, 680–8.

Kosola, S., Mundy, L. K., Sawyer, S. M., Canterford, L., van der Windt, D. A., Dunn, K. M., and Patton, G. C. (2017) Pain and learning in primary school: a population-based study. *Pain*, **158**, 1825–30.

Koutantji, M., Pearce, S. A., Oakley, D. A., and Feinmann, C. (1999) Children in pain: an investigation of selective memory for pain and psychological adjustment. *Pain*, **81**, 237–44.

Larsson, B., Carlsson, J., Fichtel, Å., and Melin, L. (2005) Relaxation treatment of adolescent headache sufferers: Results from a school-based replication series. *Headache,* **45**, 692–704.

Logan, D. E., Catanese, S. P., Coakley, R. M., and Scharff, L. (2007) Chronic pain in the classroom: Teachers' attributions about the causes of chronic pain. *Journal of School Health*, **77**, 248–56.

Logan, D. E., Coakley, R. M., and Scharff, L. (2007) Teachers' perceptions of and responses to adolescents with chronic pain syndromes. *Journal of Pediatric Psychology*, **32**, 139–49.

Logan, D. E., and Curran, J. A. (2005) Adolescent chronic pain problems in the school setting: Exploring the experiences and beliefs of selected school personnel through focus group methodology. *Journal of Adolescent Health*, **37**, 281–8.

Logan, D. E., and Scharff, L. (2005) Relationships between family and parent characteristics and functional abilities in children with recurrent pain syndromes: An investigation of moderating effects on the pathway from pain to disability. *Journal of Pediatric Psychology*, **30**, 698–707.

Logan, D. E., and Simons, L. E. (2010) Development of a group intervention to improve school functioning in adolescents with chronic pain and depressive symptoms: a study of feasibility and preliminary efficacy. *Journal of Pediatric Psychology*, **30**, 823–36.

Logan, D. E., Simons, L. E., and Carpino, E. A. (2012) Too sick for school? Parent influences on school functioning among children with chronic pain. *Pain*, **153**, 437–43.

Logan, D. E., Simons, L. E., and Kaczynski, K. J. (2009) School functioning in adolescents with chronic pain: the role of depressive symptoms in school impairment. *Journal of Pediatric Psychology*, **34**, 882–92.

Logan, D. E., Simons, L. E., Stein, M. J., and Chastain, L. (2008) School impairment in adolescents with chronic pain. *The Journal of Pain*, **9**, 407–16.

Long, A. C., Krishnamurthy, V., and Palermo, T.M. (2008) Sleep disturbances in school-age children with chronic pain. *Journal of Pediatric Psychology*, **33**, 258.

Magalnick, H., and Mazyck, D. (2008) Role of the school nurse in providing school health services. *Pediatrics*, **121**, 1052–6.

Merlijn, V. P., Hunfeld, J. A., van der Wouden, J. C., Hazebroek-Kampschreur, A. A., Koes, B. W., and Passchier, J. (2003) Psychosocial factors associated with chronic pain in adolescents. *Pain*, **101**, 33–43.

Mifflin, K., Chorney, J., and Dick, B. (2016) Attention and working memory in female adolescents with chronic pain and pain-free female adolescents: a preliminary pilot study. *The Clinical Journal of Pain*, **32**, 609–16.

Mikkelsson, M., Salminen, J. J., and Kautiainen, H. (1997) Non-specific musculoskeletal pain in preadolescents. Prevalence and 1-year persistence. *Pain*, **73**, 29–35.

Moriarty, O., McGuire, B. E., and Finn, D. P. (2011) The effect of pain on cognitive function: a review of clinical and preclinical research. *Progress in Neurobiology*, **93**, 385–404.

Reid, K., Simmonds, M., Verrier, M., and Dick, B. (2016) Supporting teens with chronic pain to obtain high school credits: Chronic Pain 35 in Alberta. *Children*, **3**, 31–42.

Rohde, G., Westergren, T., Haraldstad, K., Johannessen, B., Høie, M., Helseth, S., and Slettebø, Å. (2015) Teachers' experiences of adolescents' pain in everyday life: A qualitative study. *BMJ Open*, **5**, e007989.

Sato, A. F., Hainsworth, K. R., Khan, K. A., Ladwig, R. J., Weisman, S. J., and Davies, W. H. (2007) School absenteeism in pediatric chronic pain: Identifying lessons learned from the general school absenteeism literature. *Children's Healthcare*, **36**, 355–72.

Scales, P. C., Benson, P. L., Roehlkepartain, E. C., Sesma, Jr A., and van Dulmen, M. (2006) The role of developmental assets in predicting academic achievement: A longitudinal study. *Journal of Adolescence*, **29**, 691–708.

Shiu, S. (2001) Issues in the education of students with chronic illness. *International Journal of Disability, Development and Education*, **48**, 269–81.

Simons, L. E., Logan, D. E., Chastain, L., and Stein, M. (2010) The relation of social functioning to school impairment among adolescents with chronic pain. *The Clinical Journal of Pain*, **26**, 16–22.

Suldo, S. M., Friedrich, A. A., White, T., Farmer, J., Minch, D., and Michalowski, J. (2009) Teacher support and adolescents' subjective well-being: A mixed-methods investigation. *School Psychology Review*, **38**, 67–84.

Tarpey, S. L., Caes, L., and Heary, C. (2018) Supporting children with chronic pain in school: understanding teachers' experiences of pain in the classroom. *European Health Psychologist*, **20**, 419–24.

Vervoort, T., Logan, D. E., Goubert, L., De Clercq, B., and Hublet, A. (2014) Severity of pediatric pain in relation to school-related functioning and teacher support: An epidemiological study among school-aged children and adolescents. *Pain*, **155**, 1118–27.

Varni, J. W., Burwinkle, T. M., and Seid, M. (2006) The PedsQL 4.0 as a school population health measure: Feasibility, reliability and validity. *Quality of Life Research*, **15**, 203–15.

Walker, L. S., Claar, R. L., and Garber, J. (2002) Social consequences of children's pain: when do they encourage symptom maintenance? *Journal of Pediatric Psychology,* **27**, 689–98.

Walker, L. S., Garber, J., and Greene, J. W. (1994) Somatic complaints in pediatric patients: a prospective study of the role of negative life events, child social and academic competence, and parental somatic symptoms. *Journal of Consulting and Clinical Psychology,* **62**, 1213–21.

Walker, L. S., Guite, J. W., Duke, M., Barnard, J. A., and Greene, J. W. (1998) Recurrent abdominal pain: A potential precursor of irritable bowel syndrome in adolescents and young adults. *The Journal of Pediatrics,* **132**, 1010–15.

Walters, A. S., and Williamson, G. M. (2000) The role of activity restriction in the association between pain and depression: A study of pediatric patients with chronic pain. *Children's Health Care,* **28**, 33–50.

Zohsel, K., Hohmeister, J., Flor, H., and Hermann, C. (2008). Altered pain processing in children with migraine: An evoked potential study. *European Journal of Pain,* **12**, 1090–101.

Chapter 6

Emerging adulthood: Millennials, work, and pain

Emma Fisher and Christopher Eccleston

Introduction

'Millennials', 'Generation Y', and the pejorative 'Generation Me' have all been used to describe the generation of children, adolescents, and young people born after 1980; those emerging into adulthood in the first decade of the new millennium. Earlier generations can be broadly separated into 'Generation X', born between 1962 and 1981, and 'baby boomers', born 1946 to 1961 (Twenge et al., 2012). Generations are usually categorized by year of birth, and share life experiences at similar critical developmental periods (Kupperschmidt, 2000). Social scientists have compared these generations to better understand their characteristics, expectations, and attitudes, and how these change over time. Each cohort experiences opportunities and challenges which often define their generation. In this chapter, we will focus specifically on millennials and how they compare to earlier generations, and the relevance of those findings in the context of pain and work.

Much of the work on millennials has come from social psychology, and most of it is from WEIRD, largely North American, samples—i.e. with people from Western, Educated, Industrialized, Rich, and Democratic nations (Henrich et al., 2010). The dominant approach is a psychological one, with an interest largely in how people construct and maintain an understanding of themselves in relation to the world, and how they behave accordingly. Less common is the study of social, economic, and environmental challenges that might contribute to generationally relevant behaviour, such as changes in health, wealth, education, labour, and technology (Gratton and Scott, 2016; Hijzen et al., 2018; OECD, 2017), and how individuals, organizations, and systems might respond to these demands (e.g. in organizational leadership style (Barbuto and Gottfredson, 2016)). This work has found application in some areas of applied psychology such as occupational and educational psychology but is curiously absent from the medical or clinical psychology literatures.

When thinking about the millennial generation, there is contrasting research about their characteristics. On one hand, negative characteristics are judged to be becoming more prominent in this generation. In the USA, the dominant proponents of these views are Jean Twenge and Keith Campbell who have promoted and popularized these ideas (Campbell et al., 2015; Twenge and Campbell, 2009; Twenge et al., 2008; Twenge et al., 2012). Using population based data from the USA, they have shown that this generation is more narcissistic, selfish, and self-focused compared to earlier generations (Twenge and Campbell, 2009). For example, in 2013 Twenge wrote: 'Almost all of the empirical evidence demonstrates a rise in self focus among American young people, including narcissism, high expectations, self-esteem, thinking one is above average, and focusing on personal (vs. global) fears... The generational decreases in empathy, trust in others, civic orientation, concern for others, and attitudes toward helping the downtrodden also point toward Generation Me and away from Generation We.' (Twenge, 2013, p. 15).

Twenge argues that the relatively sudden arrival and now ubiquitous access to the Internet and its media are the major reasons for the growth in self-regard, misplaced self-belief, interest in fame for its own value, obsession with expensive material goods, and a concern for creating a perfect 'image' of oneself. Twenge (2013) does acknowledge some positives of the millennial generation, including improved acceptance of differences and increased tolerance to others. However, she considers 'narcissism' (excessive self-regard, grandiosity, and need for approbation and admiration) the defining feature of the millennial generation (Twenge et al., 2012).

Others have countered Twenge's viewpoint, arguing that millennials are less selfish, and more socially conscious than previous generations, more engaged in global and community issues (Arnett et al., 2013). Arnett and colleagues (2013) have criticized Twenge's portrayal of millennials as overly narcissistic, citing methodological problems with the databases used to monitor changes in cohort student belief over time, and a narrative over-representation of the idea of a millennial character as many of the samples also included Baby Boomers and Generation X. Curran and Hill (2019) have also found an increase in perfectionism across the millennial generation, in which people report living with high and unrealistic expectations of others, from others, and of themselves.

We are sceptical of the value of strong judgements about characteristics of whole populations. However, we recognize that there is a population of young people who have grown up in a world fundamentally different from that of previous generations, in every aspect of social, economic, technological, and health expectations and realities. In this chapter, we first provide an overview of what is known from research into the millennial generation and the world in which they exist, briefly touching on the sociological, economic, and technological context of this generation. We then discuss millennials at work, their expectations, and values in the work place. After, we turn our focus to millennials and health, how health has changed over the generations, their access to health care, and then focusing on chronic pain. We end the chapter by discussing the difficult transition from paediatric to adult services, and by providing future directions in this field.

The landscape: sociological, economic, and technology context

What makes a consideration of generational differences meaningful is to identify objective differences in the sociological, economic, technological, and health sectors that are critically different from one generation to the next. Here, we are interested in understanding differences between generations, with a specific focus on millennials, work, and pain. However, these must be considered within the social, economic, and technological context in which we live. Below is a brief summary of these. An exhaustive summary and discussion of these factors is out of our reach for this chapter but those interested could do worse than start with broad sociological, economic, and technological changes.

Sociological changes

Those born in 2015 are likely to live 12 years longer than their parents born in the 1960s (OECD Family Database, 2017). This increase in longevity is thought to be associated with a number of major demographic changes. First, attitudes to relationships and marriage have changed. Living alone, in an unmarried partnership, and raising children out of marriage are all now common. Rates of divorce of the parents of millennials are also higher, with single or blended families considered common in this generation (Kennedy and Ruggles, 2014). Second, people are also having fewer children in Western societies, meaning there is a move from having two children to one (The Statistics Portal, 2018). Educationally, in many countries children are required to stay in school until 18 years of age, and many go onto further education at colleges or universities. The development and cost of transportation has also meant for many easier and cheaper travel nationally and internationally.

Economic changes

The global economic recession of 2007 resulted in increased national debt and freezes in public sector support. An impact of this is that the millennial generation will be the first generation to be worse off compared with their parents' generation (O'Connor, 2018). In some economies, such as the UK, millennials are also the first generation to pay for higher education (Hubble and Bolton, 2018) and in the USA the cost of a university education has now reached an average of $132,860 USD (£101,505) for an undergraduate degree (Times Higher Education, 2017). Many graduates will start their working careers in significant debt. Further, in many economies, house prices have increased at a faster rate than wage increases, making home ownership an aspiration rather than the reality for many (CNCB, 2018).

Technological changes

Advancements in technology have resulted in the millennials being the first 'digital native' generation, the first to never have known life without mobile telephony and the Internet (Gray et al., 2005). Previous generations are perceived as 'digital immigrants', regardless of their knowledge of technology. The availability of technology has transformed how this generation communicates and allows for easy and often near instant access to information. However, the availability of information and instant communication can have a negative impact on individuals. Social media in particular has been criticized for the rise in mental health conditions. Bullying is no longer restricted to the playground and has resulted in increased attempted suicide in young people

(Hinduja and Patchin, 2010). Further, millennials report higher levels of social anxiety and depression associated with time spent on social media (Woods and Scott, 2016).

Millennials and work

Millennials are making up an increasing proportion of the workforce in all sectors, and at all levels. Although the media often portrays millennials as entitled, lazy, and spoilt (Hoyle, 2017), millennials are clearly motivated people. This is compounded by their high desire to progress in the work place as being the most important work-related attribute.

In a study investigating hospitality managers across three generations, millennials were found to score job switching behaviour and intention to quit higher when compared with Generation X and baby boomers (Solnet et al., 2012). These are attributes that companies would want to minimize, in order to secure a continuous workforce. In contrast, millennials rated engagement with the job, job satisfaction, and organizational commitment as low priorities compared to their earlier counterparts (Solnet et al., 2012). The social aspect of work is also important to millennials. They rated 'good people to work with' and 'good people to report to' as the second and third most desirable aspects of work (Ng et al., 2010). When splitting the millennials by age, the youngest millennials were most likely to report lower loyalty to a singular organization and rated job satisfaction, engagement, and organizational commitment as lowest compared to older millennials (Solnet et al., 2012).

As touched on already, millennials have high hopes and expectations regarding work. In a Canadian generational study, authors found millennials' expectation of a starting salary was around $43,000 in 2010 and they thought that this should increase significantly over 5 years (Ng et al., 2010). Further, two-thirds expected a promotion within 18 months of starting their first job, showing impatience and need for recognition early on (Ng et al., 2010). It is unclear how these expectations are met within the workplace, but it is likely that many are disappointed upon entering and progressing through the working sector as they fail to meet their high expectations as some work places will not be able to pay so highly or progress workers so quickly.

This disappointment has been captured in the recent discussion of what has become known as a 'quarter-life crisis'. Alan Piper argues that happiness over the life course should be considered within age cohorts and represents the dominant view that millennials are at risk of reaching an existential life-course crisis earlier than is popularly imagined in previous generations, one dominated by a subjective belief that life was not as expected and an anger at being mis-sold, misled, or deceived (Piper, 2015). Much of this work sits in the fast moving world of social media discussion, journalism, and organizational commentary, meaning it has largely escaped academic study. Because it is not studied does not mean it is unimportant. As far as we are aware there is no research or commentary on the place of pain or somatic illness in such 'crisis' episodes, or whether those episodes are characterized by psychological symptoms of mental defeat, anger, and resignation.

Kowske et al. (2010) argues that although differences exist, there are more similarities than differences, and although there might be significant differences, the effect sizes are negligible. In particular, this relates to attitudes towards satisfaction with the work itself, satisfaction with pay, and turnover intentions that although different, should be considered in terms of the small effect sizes (Kowske et al., 2010). Further, millennials' working hours are similar to Generation X's working hours, countering the impression that they work shorter days (Deal et al., 2010). Change in working patterns are traditionally thought to be driven by market need, and the direction of that change is dependent on macro-economic features such as levels of employment, speed of automation, economic migration, and wage inflation. In labour-rich markets a workforce might be expected to change their expectations to meet the demands of the job. Conversely, when employers need to compete for labour, designing work that is attractive to millennials becomes important and may involve benefits such as health care and good work–life balance (Firfiray and Mayo, 2017). Millennials may come to be considered the source of modernization of many workplaces, responsible for shaping and re-creating working practices to match new expectations, not just of work but of life.

Millennials and health

Health over the generations

Different generations and social contexts bring about different challenges for health-care systems. Currently, the most burdensome health conditions in the UK are curative and rehabilitative care, with £77.5 billion being spent in 2016 (Office for National Statistics, 2018). The greatest risk factors for both mortality and morbidity in many developed economies are cardiovascular, respiratory, and musculoskeletal, all of which are influenced by diet, tobacco and alcohol use, and lack of exercise (Barkin et al., 2010). Obesity, for example, is still rising in many countries. In the UK alone, hospital admissions where obesity was a factor increased 18% between 2015 and 2016 (National Statistics, 2018).

In addition to physical conditions, mental health conditions are also increasingly prevalent. A generational analysis identified that social economic status (SES) was a key variable in long-term mental health diagnoses. A UK study investigated the association between SES status of parents and their child's mental health during adulthood between generations (Wood et al., 2017). The authors found that children born after 1970 were more likely to report poorer mental health during adulthood if their parents had lower SES status. However, for children born before 1970, no link between SES status during childhood and later mental health was identified. This was supported by a study conducted in Germany that found an association between lower SES status and increasing chronic illness from 2003 to 2012 (Hoebel et al., 2018).

Health habits are important to consider when discussing physical and mental health of millennials. Health habits of the millennial generation are typically characterized by excessive drinking (Measham, 2008) and smoking behaviours. Although smoking in the UK has decreased since the introduction of the smoking ban in public places in 2007, millennials make up the highest proportion of smokers in the UK (Office for National Statistics, 2017). Similarly in the USA, millennials make up the highest proportion of smokers (Centers of Disease Control and Prevention, 2018). However, millennials are less likely to drink compared with their elders. In particular, around 50% of millennials report drinking in the last month compared to 65% of Generation Xers and 72% of baby boomers (Hoyer, 2017).

How Generation Y access health care

The millennial relationship with their own health, use of health care, and expectations of health care both as consumers and practitioners, is relatively unexplored. There are few research studies investigating direct comparisons of health-care use and expectations between Baby Boomers, Generation X, and Generation Y.

Health care is changing rapidly and access to health-care information is easier through mobile applications, the internet, and media. Health care has started to incorporate technology for record keeping, delivery, and assessment in many health-care delivery facilities to create a more accurate and accessible systems. For example, it is possible to have a face to face digital consultation with a health-care provider rather than in person, increasing the accessibility and flexibility of accessing health care (Fishwick, 2018). There are frequent factual as well as fictional entertainment media about mental and physical health conditions, meaning that even without actively seeking health information, we are often exposed to concepts and languages of health and illness. Similarly, we are therefore exposed to different methods of coping (adaptive, as well as maladaptive), and different treatments available.

Research on how millennials search for health-care information has been explored. In a study published in 2013 including 105 adolescents, most adolescents did not report using the internet primarily for health-care use, and few used this as a way to access health information at all. Only 14 adolescents reported searching for health-related information on the internet (Henderson et al., 2013). Of those 14 participants, most were girls. No significant differences were found on coping mechanisms when in pain or pain catastrophizing between those who sought health information online compared with those who did not.

A second study investigated how adolescents sought out young people's knowledge of health and application of health (i.e. use of health-care knowledge in real-world situations) and this was assessed across nine health areas including cancer, diabetes, HIV/AIDS, physical activity, sexuality, obesity, risk-taking behaviours, and cardiovascular health (Lloyd et al., 2013). High school students showed better understanding of applying knowledge, than having correct knowledge content. Specifically, students lacked knowledge in cancer and nutrition, but answered correctly on areas including HIV/AIDS, risky behaviours, sexuality, and obesity (Lloyd et al, 2013). However, with the rapidly evolving nature of the internet and technology-based resources, it is likely that these findings are already outdated.

Aside from the internet, the millennial generation frequently uses mobile technology and applications or 'apps'. It is estimated that children (8–15 years of age) spend between 11 and 19 hours a week online, more than double the time spent online in 2005 (Offcom, 2015). Accordingly, health information, monitoring, assessment, and treatment are available via these modes. It is also possible to track or self-monitor health behaviours through different technologies. Monitoring devices can give immediate feedback on current health status including heart rate, miles/kilometres walked, sporting exercises completed, and sleep. This feedback is continually available and can put more emphasis on the individual maintaining certain behavioural goals and reaching targets, both intrinsic and extrinsic. Whilst it is not clear how many millennials use these apps, there were 283 pain-related apps available across five app shops in December 2013 (de la Vega and Miró, 2014), which is likely to have increased. Despite these being available, none of them were designed by authors of scientific papers attempting to establish the efficacy or validity of their app. Instead, 34 pain-related apps were found through searching the scientific literature, but these were not available in stores for the general public to purchase or access. This demonstrates a disconnect between scientifically efficacious and theoretically underpinned apps that are not available publically, and those created by the non-academic community that are available to the public (de la Vega and Miró, 2014).

Finally, online social support is popular amongst the millennial generation. With easy and free access to social media platforms, online social support from friends, acquaintances, and even strangers is common and sought after. Researchers are taking advantage of such technology and connections by developing peer-support treatments (Stinson et al., 2016). This intervention paired children with juvenile idiopathic arthritis with older peers with the same condition. Older peers were provided training on conversations for mentorship calls including coping strategies, lifestyle management, communicating effectively with the health-care team. They were also provided with advice on how to structure the call. The participants in the intervention condition reported higher perceived ability to control their pain, although no differences between the peer mentoring and control group were noted for the outcomes of pain, self-efficacy, or health-related quality of life (Stinson et al., 2016).

Chronic pain in the millennial generation

Chronic pain is prevalent in children and adolescents. Prevalence studies estimate around 20–25% of children and adolescents report frequent pain (Perquin et al., 2000), lasting for longer than 3 months. For 10% of young people, this pain is disabling (Huguet and Miró, 2008). A recent definition of pain defines the experience as 'a mutually recognisable somatic experience that reflects a person's apprehension of threat to their bodily or existential integrity' (Cohen et al., 2018, p. 6), trying to capture the social and cognitive realities of pain. There are little data on how the millennial generation experience and cope with pain compared to previous generations. There is some interest in aspects of anger and disappointment at not receiving a cure (Carson et al., 2005; Pincus et al., 2018). However, there is little understanding of the broader sociological and psychological impact of being a millennial in pain.

Diagnosis and confidence in doctors when in chronic pain

Living with chronic pain can cause increased distress, disability, and reduce social functioning in young people, people emerging into adulthood (Gauntlett-Gilbert and

Eccleston, 2007, Forgeron et al., 2010, Kashikar-Zuck et al., 2008). However, the search for diagnosis can be a particularly distressing part of the patient journey. Pain is a subjective and internalized experience, which is often not associated with a visible physical injury or disease. Therefore, it can be difficult to convince others that one might be suffering and in need of succour. Particularly in western societies, labelling and providing a diagnosis, provides some validation of being 'believed' (Jordan et al., 2007). A recent topical review has highlighted this important issue in relation to children and adolescents (Pincus et al., 2018). However, little work has been conducted in children and adolescents on this construct and the implications of not being believed, not believing a diagnosis given by a medical professional, or believing that something has been missed with regards to their pain. The authors highlight the important implications diagnostic uncertainty can have for treatment, as health-care professionals are less likely to be trusted by their patients if they do not believe they have been diagnosed correctly (Pincus et al., 2018).

Research otherwise in this area is limited when considering health contexts. However, it is possible to borrow from other areas around millennial expectations towards health care. For example, in a study conducted in the hospitality sector, researchers found that millennial workers perceived their millennial line managers as more competent, compared to Baby Boomer or Generation X managers (Chi et al., 2013). This may also translate to the doctor's consultation room. Millennials may trust and feel more understood by doctors from the same generation more than other generations. Similarly, millennials are thought to be comfortable with challenging authority (Gursoy et al., 2008), and this may extend to challenging a diagnosis if they do not think that it is correct. Finally, research showing that millennials want immediate gratification, recognition, and promotion (Gursoy et al., 2013) could suggest that they want immediate tests, diagnoses, and treatment for any health conditions they experience. Some health conditions are complex, and take time to understand, diagnose, and treat. To our knowledge we do not know how millennials react or cope when faced with such situations. Whilst borrowing literature from other fields may inform hypotheses, the little research that has focused on millennials and health suggests that they are more likely to revert back to 'traditional' methods when searching for health-care information (Henderson et al., 2013), similar to their predecessors. This may also apply in the medical consultation room, throughout diagnosis, and treatment.

Although speculative, just as millennial expectations of the workplace may be a force of change in the employment sector, the same may occur in the relationship people have with medicine, health-care professionals, and health-care systems.

Impact of pain on identity

Chronic pain that persists for longer than 3 months, as well as being interruptive and interfering, can also threaten identity. Studies conducted in millennial children and adolescents who have chronic pain have begun to explore this concept. Eccleston et al. (2008) found that in a sample of children with chronic pain, they perceived themselves as further behind their healthy peers on 'independence' and 'identity formation'. Although there were no baseline data from adolescents of their perceptions of themselves before they had pain, it is clear that living with pain is associated with perceiving oneself as socially delayed (compared to their peers) on important parts of adolescence: namely emotional control and autonomy. These results were supported in a large population study including 856 adolescents with chronic pain which investigated the role of anxiety in perception of development. The authors found that higher pain-related anxiety specifically in girls, was associated with impairment in self-perception development (Caes et al., 2015). Research investigating if this perception of development recovers if pain is managed appropriately is needed, and treatments could help target these areas for millennials.

When asking about goals for the future of these young people with chronic pain, there has been relatively little prospective data collected and analysed. However, the disruptive nature of chronic pain is likely to impact the future goals of these young people which may have to change somewhat, as research shows chronic pain during childhood often persists into adulthood (Walker et al., 2010). Longitudinal studies have established that adolescents with chronic pain are less likely to get a college degree (Kashikar-Zuck et al., 2014). However, people with juvenile fibromyalgia are more likely to marry earlier, contrary to evidence that shows millennials are more likely to marry later (Kashikar-Zuck et al., 2014; Martin et al., 2014). There are no clear reasons for this difference. Other longitudinal research to investigate changes in goals when faced with adversity has not yet been conducted to our knowledge in this population. However, population-based research has been conducted and 'life goals' between baby boomers and millennials are very similar. Both generations rank 'good marriage and family' as highest, followed by steady work. Millennials then ranked 'strong friendship' and 'giving their child better opportunities' third and fourth, whilst boomers rank 'finding purpose in life' and 'strong friendships' next (Arnett et al., 2013). However, there is little understanding of the broader sociological and psychological impact of being a millennial in pain.

Transitioning into early adulthood and beyond with chronic pain

Transitioning to adulthood can be a stressful time for all adolescents, with new challenges and responsibilities, and little training in how to cope effectively with the change. There are obvious social and cultural expectations around transitioning, for example moving out of the family home, going to university, or finding work. Prevalence rates of mental health disorders often peak around this time. For example, diagnoses of depression are particularly high in early adulthood (Barth et al., 2014) and three-quarters of lifetime anxiety disorders occur before the age of 24 years (Kessler et al., 2005).

Transitioning to adulthood with a chronic pain condition brings additional challenges, particularly for people with disability who may not be able to move around as easily or quickly as their peers, or may need specific living arrangements due to their chronic pain condition. Further, chronic pain co-morbidities including higher anxiety and depressive symptoms, may result in less enthusiasm to transition, with sufferers preferring to rely on parents for an extended period of time. Most obviously, this would result in remaining in the family home and not pursuing further education or work. Parents have indeed reported an unexpected and increased burden of caring for a child with a chronic pain condition (Jordan et al., 2007).

Transferring from paediatric to adult services can be a difficult time for both patients and providers. There are many barriers to transitioning, for both the clinician or physician and the patient. These include difficulty disengaging from long-standing relationships, negative beliefs about adult care, limited knowledge of the transition process, lack of self-management skills, and financial implications (Gray et al., 2018). When considering that an adolescent may also be socially and academically behind healthy peers due to having to spend long periods of time out of school and isolated from friends, it is understandable that they may be reluctant to make the transition to adult services, when they do not consider themselves to be developmentally meeting the social and cultural targets that define adulthood.

Millennials as health-care providers

Generation Y are not only consumers of health care, but are also involved in its provision. Naturally, as each generation delivers health care, health care in turn changes. There are now more women who deliver health care. However, despite the rises of women in some professional sectors, medicine continues to be male dominated. For example, in 1965, 9% of applicants to medical colleges in the USA were female. At the cusp of the millennial generation in 1981, this percentage rose to 30%. At the turn of the millennium, 45% of applicants were female and there has been only a marginal increase to 47% in 2015 (Association of American Medical Colleges, 2016). Flexible working hours are more attainable, as parenting is a high priority for this generation.

The Institute of Medicine published their report '*To err is human*' in 1999, which reported 44,000 to 98,000 patients die annually due to medical personnel errors (Kohn et al., 1999). Millennials, along with their superiors, have endeavoured to increase the quality and safety of health care to reduce these numbers. However, in the most recent report which uses higher quality methodology compared to the 1999 report, death due to medical error is the third largest cause of death in the USA and is estimated to be 251,000 annually, much higher than predicted in 1999 (Makary and Daniel, 2016). Millennials are taking on an imperfect system in which they will face the challenges of managing an aging population. Millennials, as well as those who they treat, will have different expectations of health care, values, and habits as we have discussed previously. Their challenge will be to meet the evolving demands of those they treat, as well as of future generations.

Future directions and conclusion

Millennials are faced with challenges, different from other generations. They are driven by different motives but still share similar values. The availability and use of technology has transformed the way in which health care is delivered and can be accessed. However, we are lacking data in many areas, meaning we lack sound understanding of this generation and what differences there are between millennials and previous generations.

We propose a number of key research questions to advance this field. First, intergenerational research is needed, to truly compare attitudes across generations. There are always limits to the design of longitudinal research, not least because it is hard to predict the questions we might want to ask in the future. However, creating a databank of diverse questions and having them completed by university and non-university cohorts is a good starting point. Second, it would be interesting to investigate attitudes and behaviours towards receiving as well as providing the work of health care across generations. This knowledge is currently missing from the literature. Finally, determining how goals and expectations change when one is in pain will help us understand how individuals born in the 1980s onwards will expect their working lives to change. We are writing this chapter in 2018 and it will appear in late 2019. By 2020 more than half of the population of many countries will be millennials. And, half of the millennial populations will be adults, 18–40 years of age. In a simple way, what is unusual will become normative just with the passage of time. Although we have bemoaned the lack of research, actually all adult research will eventually be with millennials. However, if we just wait for time to pass we will miss a major opportunity to understand what we believe to be a quiet revolution in the social psychology of individuals. From the impact of perfectionism, to quarter-life crises, to the expectations of long working lives, to the emergence of the multicareers life, we need a better appreciation of how pain will experienced, can be understood, and could be managed.

References

Arnett, J. J., Trzesniewski, K. H., and Donnellan, M. B. (2013) The dangers of generational myth-making: Rejoinder to Twenge. *Emerging Adulthood,* **1**, 17–20.

Association of American Medical Colleges. (2016) Table 1. Medical students, selected years, 1965–2015. Online. Available at: https://www.aamc.org/members/gwims/statistics/gwimsstats2015-2016/ [Accessed 10th May 2018].

Barbuto, J. E., and Gottfredson, R. K. (2016) Human capital, the millennial's reign, and the need for servant leadership. *Journal of Leadership Studies,* **10**, 59–63.

Barkin, S. L., Heerman, W. J., Warren, M. D., and Rennhoff, C. (2010) Millennials and the world of work: The impact of obesity on health and productivity. *Journal of Business and Psychology,* **25**, 239–45.

Barth, J., Hofmann, K., and Schori, D. (2014) Depression in early adulthood: Prevalence and psychosocial correlates among young Swiss men. *Swiss Medical Weekly,* **144**, w13945.

Caes, L., Fisher, E., Clinch, J., Tobias, J. H., and Eccleston, C. (2015) The role of pain-related anxiety in adolescents' disability and social impairment: ALSPAC data. *European Journal of Pain,* **19**, 842–51.

Campbell, W. K., Campbell, S. M., Siedor, L. E., and Twenge, J. M. (2015) Generational differences are real and useful. *Industrial and Organizational Psychology,* **8**, 324–31.

Carson, J. W., Keefe, F. J., Goli, V., Fras, A. M., Lynch, T. R., Thorp, S. R., and Buechler, J. L. (2005) Forgiveness and chronic low back pain: A preliminary study examining the relationship of forgiveness to pain, anger, and psychological distress. *The Journal of Pain,* **6**, 84–91.

Centers of Disease Control and Prevention (2018) Current cigarette smoking among adults—United States, 2016. *Morbidity and Mortality Weekly Report* **67**, 53–9

Chi, C. G., Maier, T. A., and Gursoy, D. (2013) Employees' perceptions of younger and older managers by generation and job category. *International Journal of Hospitality Management* **34**, 42–50.

CNCB. (2018) US house prices are going to rise at twice the speed of inflation and pay: Reuters poll Online. Available at: www.cnbc.com/2018/06/06/us-house-prices-are-going-to-rise-at-twice-the-speed-of-inflation-and-pay-reuters-poll.html [Accessed 24th August 2018].

Cohen, M., Quintner, J., and Van Rysewyk, S. (2018) Reconsidering the International Association for the Study of Pain definition of pain. *Pain Reports,* **3**, e634.

Curran, T., and Hill, A. P. (2019) Perfectionism is increasing over time: a meta-analysis of birth cohort differences from 1989 to 2016. *Psychological Bulletin,* **145**, 410–29.

De La Vega, R., and Miró, J. (2014) mHealth: A strategic field without a solid scientific soul. a systematic review of pain-related apps. *PloS One,* **9**, e101312.

Deal, J. J., Altman, D. G., and Rogelberg, S. G. (2010) Millennials at work: What we know and what we need to do (if anything). *Journal of Business and Psychology,* **25**, 191–9.

Eccleston, C., Wastell, S., Crombez, G., and Jordan, A. (2008) Adolescent social development and chronic pain. *European Journal of Pain,* **12**, 765–74.

Firfiray, S., and Mayo, M. (2017) The lure of work-life benefits: Perceived person-organization fit as a mechanism explaining job seeker attraction to organizations. *Human Resource Management,* **56**, 629–49.

Fishwick, S. (2018) GP at Hand: The doctor app shaking up London's healthcare. *Evening Standard* (5 April 2018).

Forgeron, P. A., King, S., Stinson, J. N., Mcgrath, P. J., Macdonald, A. J., and Chambers, C. T. (2010) Social functioning and peer relationships in children and adolescents with chronic pain: A systematic review. *Pain Research and Management,* **15**, 27–41.

Gauntlett-Gilbert, J., and Eccleston, C. (2007) Disability in adolescents with chronic pain: Patterns and predictors across different domains of functioning. *Pain,* **131**, 132–141.

Gratton, L., and Scott, A. (2016) *The 100-Year Life: Living and Working in an Age of Longevity.* London: Bloomsbury.

Gray, N. J., Klein, J. D., Noyce, P. R., Sesselberg, T. S., and Cantrill, J. A. (2005) Health information-seeking behaviour in adolescence: the place of the internet. *Social Science & Medicine,* **60**, 1467–78.

Gray, W. N., Schaefer, M. R., Resmini-Rawlinson, A., and Wagoner, S. T. (2018) Barriers to transition from pediatric to adult care: A systematic review. *Journal of Pediatric Psychology,* **40**, 488–502.

Gursoy, D., Maier, T. A., and Chi, C. G. (2008) Generational differences: An examination of work values and generational gaps in the hospitality workforce. *International Journal of Hospitality Management,* **27**, 448–58.

Gursoy, G., Chi, C. G., and Karadag, E. (2013) Generational differences in work values and attitudes among frontline and service contact employees. *International Journal of Hospitality Management,* **32**, 40–8.

Henderson, E. M., Keogh, E., Rosser, B. A., and Eccleston, C. (2013) Searching the Internet for help with pain: Adolescent search, coping, and medication behaviour. *British Journal of Health Psychology,* **18**, 218–32.

Henrich, J., Heine, S. J., and Norenzayan, A. (2010) The weirdest people in the world? *Behavioral & Brain Sciences,* **33**, 61–83; discussion 83–135.

Hijzen, A., Kappeler, A., Pak, M., and Schwellnus, C. (2018) Labour market resilience: The role of structural and macroeconomic policies. In: de Haan, J., and Parlevliet, J. (eds) *Structural Reforms*. Cham: Springer, 173–98.

Hinduja, S., and Patchin, J. W. (2010) Bullying, cyberbullying, and suicide. *Archives of Suicide Research*, **14**, 206–21.

Hoebel, J., Kuntz, B., Moor, I., Kroll, L. E., and Lampert, T. (2018) Post-millennial trends of socioeconomic inequalities in chronic illness among adults in Germany. *BMC Research Notes*, **11**, 200.

Hoyer, H. (2017) Millennials think before they drink: Fewer rounds, less carbs, more variety. Online. Available at: http://www.nielsen.com/au/en/insights/news/2017/millennials-think-before-they-drink-fewer-rounds-less-carbs-more-variety.html. [Accessed 26th July 2018]

Hoyle, A. (2017) A generation with a huge sense of entitlement: Bosses complain that Millennials are spoilt, full of themselves, averse to hard work and expect 'success on a plate' so what does that mean for society? *Daily Mail* (16 February 2017).

Hubble, S., and Bolton, P. (2018) Higher education tuition fees in England. House of Commons Library. Briefing Paper Number 8151.

Huguet, A. and Miró, J. (2008) The severity of chronic pediatric pain: an epidemiological study. *The Journal of Pain*, **9**, 226–36.

Jordan, A. L., Eccleston, C., and Osborn, M. (2007) Being a parent of the adolescent with complex chronic pain: An interpretative phenomenological analysis. *European Journal of Pain*, **11**, 49–56.

Kashikar-Zuck, S., Cunningham, N., Sil, S., Bromberg, M. H., Lynch-Jordan, A. M., Strotman, D., et al. (2014) Long-term outcomes of adolescents with juvenile-onset fibromyalgia in early adulthood. *Pediatrics*, **133**, e592–600.

Kashikar-Zuck, S., Parkins, I. S., Graham, T. B., Lynch, A. M., Passo, M., Johnston, M., et al. (2008) Anxiety, mood, and behavioral disorders among pediatric patients with juvenile fibromyalgia syndrome. *The Clinical Journal of Pain*, **24**, 620–6.

Kennedy, S., and Ruggles, S. (2014) Breaking up is hard to count: the rise of divorce in the United States, 1980–2010. *Demography*, **51**, 587–98.

Kessler, R. C., Berglund, P., Demler, O., Jin, R., Merikangas, K. R., and Walters, E. E. (2005) Lifetime prevalence and age-of-onset distributions of DSM-IV disorders in the National Comorbidity Survey Replication. *Archives of General Psychiatry*, **62**, 593–602.

Kohn, K. T., Corrigan, J. M., and Donaldson, M. S. (1999) *To Err Is Human: Building a Safer Health Care System*. Washington, DC: National Academy Press.

Kowske, B. J., Rasch, R., and Wiley, J. (2010) Millennials' (lack of) attitude problem: An empirical examination of generational effects on work attitudes. *Journal of Business and Psychology*, **25**, 265–79.

Kupperschmidt, B. R (2000) Multigeneration employees: strategies for effective management. *The Health Care Manager*, **19**, 65–76.

Lloyd, T., Shaffer, M. L., Christy, S., Widome, M. D., Repke, J., Weitekamp, M. R., et al. (2013) Health knowledge among the millennial generation. *Journal of Public Health Research*, **2**, 38.

Makary, M. A., and Daniel, M. (2016) Medical error-the third leading cause of death in the US. *BMJ: British Medical Journal (Online)*, **353**: i2139.

Martin, S. P., Astone, N. M., and Peters, H. E. (2014) Fewer marriages, more divergence: marriage projections for millennials to age 40. Urban Institute. Online. Available at: https://www.urban.org/research/publication/

fewer-marriages-more-divergence-marriage-projections-millennials-age-40 [Accessed August 2018].

Measham, F. (2008) The turning tides of intoxication: young people's drinking in Britain in the 2000s. *Health Education,* **108**, 207–22.

National Statistics. (2018) Statistics on obesity, diet, and physical activity. England 2018. Online. Available at: https://digital.nhs.uk/data-and-information/publications/statistical/statistics-on-obesity-physical-activity-and-diet/statistics-on-obesity-physical-activity-and-diet-england-2018 [Accessed 24th August 2018].

Ng, E. S., Schweitzer, L., and Lyons, S. T. (2010) New generation, great expectations: A field study of the millennial generation. *Journal of Business and Psychology,* **25**, 281–92.

O'Connor, S. (2018) Millennials poorer than previous generations, data shows. *Financial Times* (23 February 2018).

OECD (2017) *Education at a Glance 2017: OECD Indicators.* Paris: OECD Publishing.

OECD Family Database (2017) Co1.2: Life expectancy at birth.

Ofcom. (2015) Children and parents: Media use and attitudes report. Online. Available at: https://www.ofcom.org.uk/__data/assets/pdf_file/0024/78513/childrens_parents_nov2015.pdf [Accessed 10th May 2018].

Office for National Statistics. (2017) Adult smoking habits in the UK: 2017. Online. Available at: https://www.ons.gov.uk/peoplepopulationandcommunity/healthandsocialcare/healthandlifeexpectancies/bulletins/adultsmokinghabitsingreatbritain/2017 -characteristics-of-current-cigarette-smokers-in-the-uk. [Accessed 26th July 2018]

Office for National Statistics (2018) UK Health Accounts: 2016. Online. Available at: https://www.ons.gov.uk/peoplepopulationandcommunity/healthandsocialcare/healthcaresystem/bulletins/ukhealthaccounts/2016 [Accessed 26th July 2018].

Perquin, C. W., Hazebroek-Kampschreur, A. A. J. M., Hunfeld, J. A., Bohnen, A. M., Van Suijlekom-Smit, L. W. A., Passchier, J., and Van Der Wouden, J. C. (2000) Pain in children and adolescents: a common experience. *Pain,* **87**, 51–8.

Pincus, T., Noel, M., Jordan, A., and Serbic, D. (2018) Perceived diagnostic uncertainty in pediatric chronic pain. *Pain,* **159**, 1198–201.

Piper, A. T. (2015) Sliding down the U-shape? A dynamic panel investigation of the age-well-being relationship, focusing on young adults. *Social Science & Medicine,* **143**, 54–61.

Solnet, D., Kralj, A., and Kandampully, J. (2012) Generation Y employees: An examination of work attitude differences. *Journal of Applied Management and Entrepreneurship,* **17**, 36–54.

Stinson, J. N., Ahola Kohut, S., Forgeron, P., Amaria, K., Bell, M., Kaufman, M., et al. (2016) The iPeer2Peer Program: a pilot randomized controlled trial in adolescents with Juvenile Idiopathic Arthritis. *Pediatric Pheumatology Online Journal,* **14**, 48.

The Statistics Portal. (2018) The average number of people per family in the United States from 1960 to 2017. Online. Available at: www.statista.com/statistics/183657/average-size-of-a-family-in-the-us [Accessed 23rd August 2018].

Times Higher Education. (2017) The cost of studying at a university in the United States. Online. Available at: https://www.timeshighereducation.com/student/advice/cost-studying-university-united-states

Twenge, J. M. (2013) The evidence for Generation Me and against Generation We. *Emerging Adulthood,* **1**, 11–16.

Twenge, J. M., and Campbell, W. K. (2009) *The Narcissism Epidemic: Living in the Age of Entitlement.* Simon and Schuster: New York.

Twenge, J. M., Campbell, W. K., and Freeman, E. C. (2012) Generational differences in young adults' life goals, concern for others, and civic orientation, 1966–2009. *Journal of Personality and Social Psychology*, **102**, 1045–62.

Twenge, J. M., Konrath, S., Foster, J. D., Campbell, W. K., and Bushman, B. J. (2008) Egos inflating over time: a cross-temporal meta-analysis of the Narcissistic Personality Inventory. *Journal of Personality*, **76**, 875–902; discussion 903–28.

Walker, L. S., Dengler-Crish, C. M., Rippel, S., and Bruehl, S. (2010) Functional abdominal pain in childhood and adolescence increases risk for chronic pain in adulthood. *Pain*, **150**, 568–72.

Wood, N., Bann, D., Hardy, R., Gale, C., Goodman, A., Crawford, C., and Stafford, M. (2017) Childhood socioeconomic position and adult mental wellbeing: Evidence from four British birth cohort studies. *PloS One*, **12**, e0185798.

Woods, H. C., and Scott, H. (2016) #Sleepyteens: social media use in adolescence is associated with poor sleep quality, anxiety, depression and low self-esteem. *Journal of Adolescence*, **51**, 41–9.

Chapter 7

Workers with occupational pain

Jos Verbeek

Introduction

The traditional world of work is explored, in particular how the changing patterns of work outlined in Chapter 2, such as the rise of mechanization, of emotional labour, and changing expectations of work, affect first how people and organizations respond to pain in the workforce, and second how the workforce of pain management specialists is responding. Occupational pain is defined as pain that is caused by occupational activities. This additional diagnosis of occupational origin is important for pain management, prevention, and compensation.

The definition of occupational pain as that caused by occupational activities is very similar to the definition of occupational disease as a disease that is wholly or partially caused by work or working conditions. A more encompassing definition is work-related disease which also includes diseases that are aggravated by work. A good example is occupational asthma that can be caused by, for example, exposure to diisocyanates[1] at work and aggravated by exposure to second-hand smoke that will worsen the symptoms (Verbeek, 2012).

Occupational pain is not a term that is used much in the literature. This is because most occupational pain is musculoskeletal and this is named according to its specific location or an assumed causal mechanism, such as occupational back pain or cumulative trauma injury. There are also other occupational pain syndromes that are not in the musculoskeletal system, such as cranial neuralgia caused by helmets (Chalela, 2018). However, this is an exception. Here, I will use occupational pain as an umbrella term to cover all pain that is somehow related to work or occupational activities. The adjective occupational is what makes the term different from pain as a diagnosis as such. This is important because the occupational origin of pain has implications for therapy, prevention, and financial compensation.

The history of occupational pain is long. As long ago as 1700, Ramazzini recognized that occupations that required awkward postures, repetitive movements, and lifting heavy weights could lead to musculoskeletal pain (Franco, 1999). There has been little change in this concept since then with the focus of research and management completely on the origins of pain in work or working conditions. This has led to a preventive practice, where tasks and jobs are designed to make them compatible with the needs, abilities, and limitations of people and thus prevent occupational pain.

---

[1] One of a family of chemicals known to cause occupational asthma and dermal problems

---

Box 7.1 A worker with occupational pain

John Doe is a 45-year-old dental hygienist whose main task is to remove plaque from the client's teeth. He has been doing this for 25 years in a small co-operative practice of five dentists and five dental hygienists. For a couple of months, he has had a nagging pain in the right arm and shoulder especially when working with patients, and the pain also keeps him awake at night. This is the first time this has occurred. Otherwise he is healthy and physically fit. There are no other problems in the workplace except that the client load that has recently increased considerably.

John sees his general practitioner for his pain. She examines the shoulder and tells him that there is no specific cause for the shoulder or the arm pain and advises him to take it easy and not to overload the arm. She also advises him to take a simple analgesic at six hourly intervals. Because John does not have any improvement, he calls in sick and stays at home where after 2 weeks the pain gradually diminishes. However, on returning to work, after 2 days of work the pain resumes and so John stops working.

The dental clinic does not have connections to an occupational health service but John's supervisor is aware of ergonomic risks in dental practice and hires a physiotherapist to check the workplace for adverse ergonomic factors. The physiotherapist advises that John should have a better posture at work with less elevation of the shoulders. The advice is also to improve the grip and to widen the diameter of the scaling instruments as this will decrease the passive force needed to hold them. It is expected that these workplace improvements will decrease the arm and shoulder pain.

In the management of patients with occupational pain, in the past, there has been little attention paid to how to keep them in the workforce. Only more recently, as a result of the advocacy of Waddell (2004) and later Black (2008) in the UK, the focus of occupational pain shifted to return to work of pain patients and to enabling work participation for patients with pain.

I will first describe a case of occupational pain and then discuss the implications that an additional diagnosis of occupational origin has for therapy, prevention, and compensation.

A diagnosis of occupational pain

In the case described in Box 7.1, the supervisor made an implicit diagnosis of occupational pain that resulted in an important shift of management. Instead of focusing on pain relief through medication and rest, workplace improvements were proposed.

I will explain how you can make an additional diagnosis of occupational origin of the pain even though this will not be easy in an individual. There are four elements that are important for such a diagnosis (Box 7.2) (Verbeek, 2012). First there has to be a clear diagnosis of the pain; then there has to be an assessment that there has been

Box 7.2 Diagnosis of occupational origin of pain

Diagnosis of occupational origin of pain should be based on

1. Diagnosis of pain referring to causal structures
2. Assessment of exposure that would lead to overload of musculoskeletal or other structures
3. Evidence in a systematic review of the relation between exposure and pain
4. Evidence that no other confounding factors can explain this relationship

Source: data from Verbeek J. (2012). When Work Is Related to Disease, What Establishes Evidence for a Causal Relation? *Saf Health Work* 3(2):110–6. https://doi.org/10.5491/Shaw.2012.3.2.110.

sufficient exposure to a causal agent at work such as an overload of the specific musculoskeletal structure to which the pain is ascribed; next there has to be evidence that there is a relationship between these two; and finally there should preferably be no other factors that can cause the pain.

A focused medical examination of the shoulder and the arm could lead to a specific diagnosis such as osteoarthritis of the shoulder joint. However, most musculoskeletal pain is non-specific and cannot be defined other than as non-specific shoulder pain (Miranda et al., 2005). Then it will be useful to have a clear subjective assessment of the pain intensity with a Visual Analogue Scale (VAS) and the disability with the DASH questionnaire (Angst et al., 2011). This can be used for evaluation of the development of the pain over time and to assess the effects of possible interventions. It is good to note that surveys of work-related pain often report only mild pain ratings. Even though such pain can be annoying and decrease quality of life, patients consider the impact of severe pain on their quality of life as much more serious. On the other hand, it is also clear that chronic pain has a profound impact on work participation (Patel et al., 2012).

The objective assessment of overloading biomechanical factors in the work situation depends on the measurement of forces, postures, and movements. These can be objectively measured but that is technically not easy and one needs specific instruments such as inclinometers and accelerometers (Trask et al., 2014). Simple assessments based on observations exist but their validity has not been assessed thoroughly (Takala et al., 2010).

The evidence for the relationship between adverse ergonomic factors and pain should come from a good systematic review from cohort studies that takes into account the factors that can confound the relationship. There is good evidence that shoulder complaints can be related to the work situation (van der Windt et al., 2000). For the pain problem in dentists, there are no good systematic reviews available even though reports of prevalence of pain suggest that there is a substantial problem (Hayes et al., 2009). Many reviews are based on cross-sectional studies or include cross-sectional studies that do not provide good evidence for a causal relationship. There are many reports available of cross-sectional studies because it is so easy to ask workers about pain and adverse biomechanical factors at the same time. In these studies, it is impossible to make a distinction between factors that worsen the pain and factors that cause the pain, because there is no temporal relationship between exposure and outcome.

There are many factors that can confound the relation between exposure at work and pain such as age and recreational activities. Pain resulting from musculoskeletal degeneration, such as the tendon of the biceps muscle, occurs much more frequently in workers above the age of 45. Since age and cumulative exposure are closely related, it is difficult to disentangle these factors. Even though non-occupational pain will be as annoying for a worker as occupational pain, the important difference is that workplace changes probably won't be effective.

Interventions for occupational pain

When a clear diagnosis of occupational pain is established, one would like to see evidence that specific ergonomic improvements help to alleviate the pain. Even though there are many studies that propose ergonomic improvements, there are only a few studies that have evaluated the effects of interventions on pain. For example, incorrect lifting techniques are often implicated as the cause of back pain. However, there are no studies that have evaluated the effect of training in correct lifting techniques for patients with existing back pain (Verbeek et al., 2012). For another frequently occurring pain resulting from the upper limb, there were 13 studies that evaluated various ergonomic interventions. The interventions did not lead to a consistent beneficial effect on pain (Verhagen et al., 2013).

The distinction between treatment and prevention is difficult in studies that include workers exposed to factors that can result in pain. If we define prevention as an intervention provided to healthy persons without the condition at hand, it will be very difficult to find participants because pain is so common that there will always be a proportion of participants that are in pain. I also consider it important to distinguish between an intervention delivered at the patient's request, as usually is the case in a treatment situation, and an intervention not delivered at the patient's behest but rather offered by the provider as part of prevention. Treatment would be easier to define as an intervention that is delivered at the request of the patient. However, randomized studies of such a treatment intervention are not available.

In the case of our dental hygienist, there is one randomized controlled trial (RCT) that answers the question if in dental hygienists, exposed to biomechanical factors overloading musculoskeletal structures, better-designed scaling instruments will decrease pain in the shoulder, elbow, or hand (Rempel et al., 2012). This study impresses as a well-designed trial. The intervention consists of a redesigned scaling instrument which has been made lighter and wider. This decreases the forces needed to hold it and also the static forces on the rest of the upper limb. The average pain level measured at baseline in the study was 2.0 ± 2.0 (mean (M) ± standard deviation (SD)) on a 10-point VAS-scale. The intervention group had a statistically significant decrease of 0.3 score points in right shoulder pain measured on the 10-point VAS-scale. It is not easy to translate these findings to our patient. First, the average level of pain at the start of the study is quite low and would be considered mild pain at best. Then, the average change in pain of 0.3 on a 10-point scale is not clinically relevant for a pain patient. Pain patients expect a treatment to lead to at least a 50% decrease in pain levels or a return to mild pain levels (O'Brien et al., 2010). Therefore, in clinical terms, the average results of this trial are not relevant for our patient. The authors considered the trial as a trial of prevention and not of management. However, there are no trials that use ergonomics as part of the management of pain in dental staff. All available trials offer the intervention to all employees who are at work and have varying, usually mild, levels of pain on average. Based on this study, it could be worthwhile to give the ergonomic intervention a try, but it is difficult to predict if there would be a beneficial effect.

Prevention of occupational pain

In many occupations, situations occur in which there is biomechanical overload such as in the case of the dental hygienist where excessive force is needed to hold instruments. Thus, it would be obvious to use the intervention to decrease these forces for all workers by using lighter instruments that are better to grasp and hold and thus prevent the resulting occupational pain. This approach has been applied to work situations and tools in many occupations and has certainly decreased force and physical exertion and improved comfort. The back is one of the most frequent anatomical sources of occupational pain. It provides a good example of efforts to prevent pain through ergonomic measures. There is, what I would qualify as modest, evidence that lifting heavy loads leads to more back pain. A systematic review of individual patient data of 220 studies on biomechanical exposure and back pain found small to moderate Odds Ratios (OR) (ranging from 1.1 to 2.1) for the association of mechanical exposures and low back pain and concluded that the relationships were complex (Griffith et al., 2012). The review did specifically not find a dose–exposure relationship. Another more recent review of occupational lifting and carrying also found a relation with lumbosacral neuropathy but did not include back pain (Kuijer et al., 2018). All in all, there seems to be some evidence for an occupational origin of back pain in workers.

One of the oldest approaches to preventing occupational back pain is to teach workers a specific posture in which to lift loads manually. The idea is that keeping the back straight and not bending or twisting the back will diminish the forces on the lower back. This will then result in less noticed or unnoticed damage to the cartilage and other spinal structures and this would also result in less pain. It is unclear where the origin of this idea lies but it was certainly enhanced by the discovery of the protruded or slipped inter-vertebral disc in 1933 by Mixter and Barr (1934). These neurosurgeons were the first to operate on a patient with back pain and find that the inter-vertebral disc was the cause of the back pain. They concluded that such a slipped disc could only be the result of an injury and since then the concept of a back injury has been used. Back pain was regarded as an early symptom of the radiating pain typical for a damaged disc. This resulted in treatments such as a plaster-jacket to keep the back straight and give rest to the disc so that it could heal (Crisp, 1945). This was also extended to prevention, where the straight back would prevent the slipping of the disc and thus also prevent back pain.

Keeping the back straight while lifting loads from a lower level is only possible by bending the knees. Therefore, this is called the squat lift as opposed to a stoop lift in which the back is bent forward. Even though it is argued that the biomechanical forces on the back are not less while using the squat lift compared with the stoop lift (van Dieen et al., 1999), this provides for an interesting intervention that can be evaluated in practice. A systematic review of interventions that trained workers to lift correctly yielded nine RCTs and nine cohort studies with in total more than 20 000 participants and conducted over a period ranging from 1981 to 2010 (Verbeek et al., 2012). None of the studies showed a statistically significant beneficial result of the training. As many participants in the intervention groups as in the control groups experienced back pain during follow up, which was as extensive as 5 years in one included study (Daltroy et al., 1997). The intervention was very intensive in one study with biofeedback devices to indicate incorrect lifting and extensive on the job training (Lavender et al., 2007). Some of the studies included in the review also measured if it was possible to make workers change their lifting behaviour. Even though there was some change, this was only small and was unlikely to lead to substantially lighter loads on the back (Lavender et al., 2007). Also none of the meta-analyses in the review yielded a significant effect. In general, it is difficult to establish that there is no effect of an intervention since even small effects can be relevant in some situations. Because so many people lift and so many experience back pain, even very small preventive effects can result in prevention of back pain in many thousands of people in a population. Even though the results of the review cannot rule out very small preventive effects, the studies needed to show such effects would have to have a very large number of participants. It is unrealistic to expect that these will ever be realized in workers. This leads me to conclude that training workers in correct lifting techniques is not an effective intervention.

The belief that a straight back is important in preventing back pain and that ergonomic measures are needed is historically deeply rooted and apparently difficult to change. One of the reasons why change is difficult is that many of these preventive ideas are laid down in regulations. For example, the EU directive on the safety requirements for the manual handling of loads stipulates: 'employers must ensure that workers receive in addition proper training and information on how to handle loads correctly and the risks they might be open to particularly if these tasks are not performed correctly' (EU-OSHA, 2019). Unfortunately, there is no intention to make changes to this regulation. This is due to the way health and safety at work is regulated. In Europe, this is based on tri-partite discussions between policy makers, trade-unions, and employers. There is no role for scientific evidence in this process. A trade-union representative once explained to me that even though it might not work, it is still an achievement of our negotiations and therefore should stay.

Training of workers is just one approach to the prevention of back pain. There are many other approaches that more directly target the work load. Lightening the load of lifting is an obvious alternative. This can be done by providing aids or tools to assist workers or by decreasing the frequency with which they have to lift. There are no studies that indicate that this will have a beneficial effect on back pain, but there are studies that can show if the biomechanical load is less with these measures. Based on evidence for decreasing load on the back, Kuijer et al. (2014) recommended use of patient lifting devices and lifting devices for goods, optimizing working height, and reducing load mass. However, future studies should also evaluate if this leads to a decrease in back pain.

Occupational pain in the upper limb is another occupational pain site which occurs frequently and which has been studied well. From music and sports, pain in the upper limb was known as overuse syndrome and ascribed to repeated exposure to awkward postures or repetitive movements. With the advent of computers in the 1980s and 1990s, the first prototypes of keyboards and screens were clumsy and not well adapted to be good human–machine interfaces. This led to discomfort and pain, while working with computers. At that time, there were no programmes that could easily enter data into the machines and most of it had to be done by people. Entering data during most of the day with clumsy equipment led almost inevitably to postures and movements that caused overload on the musculoskeletal system which was named repetitive strain injury (RSI) or cumulative trauma disorder. Basically this referred to pain in the hand, arm, or shoulder that was ascribed to working with the computer. In the USA the syndrome was named cumulative trauma disorder with a similar idea that repetition of movement can lead to trauma in musculoskeletal structures leading to inflammation and pain. For some musculoskeletal disorders, such as De Quervain's tenosynovitis,[2] it had been recognized that force and repetition could play a causal role in inflammation of the sheath of the tendons of the thumb even though more recently this was not confirmed in a systematic review (Stahl et al., 2013). Similarly, carpal tunnel syndrome was ascribed to repetitive work already before computers had arrived to the world of work. However, with the advent of computers non-specific pain of the upper limb was also diagnosed as occupational. This led to hot debate and controversies about the usefulness of this extra diagnosis of occupational origin. Those that had to manage the pain of these patients felt that an occupational diagnosis hindered rehabilitation and led to more frequent disability. On the other hand, those that were in favour of preventive interventions felt that even if only a part of the occupational upper limb pain is caused by occupational factors it would be ergonomics that would help to prevent pain in still a considerable number of people.

A Cochrane review of ergonomic interventions for preventing work-related musculoskeletal disorders of the upper limb and neck among office workers found 15 RCTs with 2165 workers that evaluated physical changes in the computer environment, different types of breaks and training of workers (Hoe et al., 2012). The authors concluded that physical changes had an inconsistent effect on pain or disability. For breaks and training they found only single studies with very low quality evidence of an effect.

It is not very clear whether these results should be interpreted as a lack of an effect of ergonomic interventions in computer work. In the past 30 years enormous improvements have been made to the human–machine interfaces for computers and many of the ergonomic problems that existed in the beginning have been resolved. The keyboards are slim and the visibility on the screen has improved enormously. This is something that the trials in the review didn't capture simply because these changes

---

[2] A tenosynovitis is a condition in which the tendons and the sheaths in which the tendons move are inflamed causing pain and impaired function.

have not been tested in RCTs and are implemented already on a wide scale. At the same time, it seems that the diagnosis of occupational upper limb disorders is in decline even though it is difficult to find good figures to underpin this. As an illustration of the possible decline, I found figures at the Dutch Centre for Occupational Diseases that reported 1257 cases of RSI in 2005 but only 68 in 2016 (NCvB 2019).

Compensation for occupational pain

Another consequence of the extra diagnosis of the occupational origin of pain is that a worker can ask for compensation for the financial losses resulting from their disorder from the employer. Criteria for financial compensation are very much dependent on national policies and on insurance policies. For example, in the Netherlands, there is very little focus on financial compensation for occupational disease. The reason for this is that there is a no-fault comprehensive wage loss compensation system in the case of disability, and full coverage of health insurance. In other countries, wage loss compensation and health benefits are only paid if the injury or disease can be ascribed to an occupational origin.

Historically, financial compensation has been a major driver of ascribing specific causes to an injury or disease. For example, financial compensation for back pain was a hot issue with the introduction of railways in the nineteenth century. Because the speed of the trains was comparatively high and many accidents occurred, back pain in people involved in such accidents was considered to result from an injured spine called a 'railway spine'. People with this disorder could sue the railway company for financial compensation which led to debates about the origins of the back pain. In general, the relation with the exposure to the train accidents was not considered very plausible and at the beginning of the twentieth century the term 'railway spine' gradually disappeared.

Whichever way workers are financially compensated, the costs of long-term disability and unemployment resulting from occupational pain are substantial. In the latest Global Burden of Disease estimate, low back pain was the leading cause of disability in the world (Global Burden of Disease Cancer et al., 2017). Cost of illness studies that have included the indirect costs of lost work productivity as a result of back pain disability report that these costs presented the majority of the total costs (Dagenais et al., 2008). Even when only a small amount of back pain can be diagnosed as being occupational, disability resulting from occupational back pain will be substantial. This is a major driver for finding effective return-to-work interventions for persons who are disabled as a result of pain. However, this is not a problem that is specific to occupational pain but one that affects all persons with pain and resulting disability (Patel et al., 2012).

Future research

We need a better understanding of whether ergonomic interventions have an effect on occupational pain as part of the treatment of pain patients. Therefore, we need RCTs that include patients with relatively high levels of occupational pain. To better understand the effects of preventive studies, we need studies with a large number of participants. This is because only then can we reliably demonstrate small effects that can still be interesting from a preventive point of view.

To make studies more comparable, researchers need to work towards consensus about the outcomes that should be used in such trials and how to measure them. For pain measurements these are available but not for disability and work participation. Funders and journals should make the use of these outcomes mandatory.

Regulation in the EU that mandates specific ergonomic or other workplace requirements should be evaluated against the state of the art in science. For future regulation, the EU should include scientific evidence to underpin the effectiveness of the interventions mandated by the regulation. With changes in the workplace and advanced knowledge of specific risks, the regulation should be flexible enough to adapt to progressing science.

Conclusions

Occupational pain is pain in which the causes are ascribed to work or working conditions. The added diagnosis of occupational origin can be important for therapy, prevention, and compensation. At an individual level, the diagnosis of occupational pain is complicated because most pain does not result from a well-defined disease and there are many confounding factors. Only if there is a clear diagnosis of an occupational origin, can it be expected that ergonomic interventions will have an effect. For prevention, ergonomic interventions can theoretically be more effective even if the occupational origin of pain is less clear. However, evaluation studies do not really confirm this. Financial compensation for losses that result from the pain has been an important driver for finding occupational causes of the pain. In the past, compensation for loss caused by pain has been related to the introduction of new technology, such as railways or computers. However, over time opinions on the occupational origin of pain have often changed. Current research is more driven by the financial impact of disability resulting from pain than by the occupational causes.

References

Angst, F., Schwyzer, H. K., Aeschlimann, A., Simmen, B. R., and Goldhahn, J. (2011) Measures of adult shoulder function: Disabilities of the Arm, Shoulder, and Hand Questionnaire (DASH) and its short version (QuickDASH), Shoulder Pain and Disability Index (SPADI), American Shoulder and Elbow Surgeons (ASES) Society standardized shoulder assessment form, Constant (Murley) Score (CS), Simple Shoulder Test (SST), Oxford Shoulder Score (OSS), Shoulder Disability Questionnaire (SDQ), and Western Ontario Shoulder Instability Index (WOSI). *Arthritis Care Research (Hoboken)*, **63** Suppl 11, S174–88.

Black, C. (2008) *Working for a Healthier Tomorrow*. London: The Stationary Office.

Chalela, J. A. (2018) Helmet-induced occipital neuralgia in a military aviator. *Aerospace Medicine and Human Performance*, **89**, 409–10.

Crisp, E. J. (1945) Damaged intervertebral disk early diagnosis and treatment. *Lancet*, **246**, 422–3.

Dagenais, S., Caro, J., and **Haldeman, S.** (2008) A systematic review of low back pain cost of illness studies in the United States and internationally. *Spine Journal,* **8,** 8–20.

Daltroy, L. H., Iversen, M. D., Larson, M. G., Lew, R., Wright, E., Ryan, J., et al. (1997) A controlled trial of an educational program to prevent low back injuries. *New England Journal of Medicine,* **337,** 322–8.

European Agency for Safety and Health at Work (Eu-Osha). (2019) *Directive 90/269/Eec— manual handling of loads.* Online. Available at: https://osha.europa.eu/en/legislation/ directives/6 [Accessed 9th April 2019].

Franco, G. (1999) Ramazzini and workers' health. *Lancet,* **354,** 858–61.

Global Burden of Disease Cancer Collaboration, Fitzmaurice, C., Allen, C., Barber, R. M., Barregard, L., Bhutta, Z. A., et al. (2017) Global, regional, and national cancer incidence, mortality, years of life lost, years lived with disability, and disability-adjusted life-years for 32 cancer groups, 1990 to 2015: a systematic analysis for the global burden of disease study. *JAMA Oncology,* **3,** 524–48.

Griffith, L. E., Shannon, H. S., Wells, R. P., Walter, S. D., Cole, D. C., Cote, P., et al. (2012) Individual participant data meta-analysis of mechanical workplace risk factors and low back pain. *American Journal of Public Health,* **102,** 309–18.

Hayes, M., Cockrell, D., and **Smith, D. R.** (2009) A systematic review of musculoskeletal disorders among dental professionals. *International Journal of Dental Hygiene,* **7,** 159–65.

Hoe, V. C., Urquhart, D. M., Kelsall, H. L., and **Sim, M. R.** (2012) Ergonomic design and training for preventing work-related musculoskeletal disorders of the upper limb and neck in adults. *Cochrane Database Systematic Review,* Cd008570.

Kuijer, P., Verbeek, J. H., Seidler, A., Ellegast, R., Hulshof, C. T. J., Frings-Dresen, M. H. W., and **Van Der Molen, H. F.** (2018) Work-relatedness of lumbosacral radiculopathy syndrome: review and dose-response meta-analysis. *Neurology,* **91,** 558–64.

Kuijer, P. P., Verbeek, J. H., Visser, B., Elders, L. A., Van Roden, N., Van Den Wittenboer, M. E., et al. (2014) An evidence-based multidisciplinary practice guideline to reduce the workload due to lifting for preventing work-related low back pain. *Annals of Occupational and Environmental Medicine,* **26,** 16.

Lavender, S. A., Lorenz, E. P., and **Andersson, G. B.** (2007) Can a new behaviorally oriented training process to improve lifting technique prevent occupationally related back injuries due to lifting? *Spine (Phila Pa 1976),* **32,** 487–94.

Miranda, H., Viikari-Juntura, E., Heistaro, S., Heliovaara, M., and **Riihimaki, H.** (2005) A population study on differences in the determinants of a specific shoulder disorder versus nonspecific shoulder pain without clinical findings. *American Journal of Epidemiology,* **161,** 847–55.

Mixter, W. J., and **Barr, J. S.** (1934) Rupture of the intervertebral disk with involvement of the spinal canal. *New England Journal of Medicine,* **211,** 210–15.

Netherlands Center for Occupational Diseases (NCvB). (2019) Online. Available at: www. beroepsziekten.nl (Dutch) or https://www.occupationaldiseases.nl/ (English).

O'Brien, E. M., Staud, R. M., Hassinger, A. D., Mcculloch, R. C., Craggs, J. G., Atchison, J. W., Price, D. D., and **Robinson, M. E.** (2010) Patient-centered perspective on treatment outcomes in chronic pain. *Pain Medicine,* **11,** 6–15.

Patel, A. S., Farquharson, R., Carroll, D., Moore, A., Phillips, C. J., Taylor, R. S., and **Barden, J.** (2012) The impact and burden of chronic pain in the workplace: a qualitative systematic review. *Pain Practice,* **12,** 578–89.

Rempel, D., Lee, D. L., Dawson, K., and Loomer, P. (2012) The effects of periodontal curette handle weight and diameter on arm pain: a four-month randomized controlled trial. *Journal of American Dental Association,* **143,** 1105–13.

Stahl, S., Vida, D., Meisner, C., Lotter, O., Rothenberger, J., Schaller, H. E., and Stahl, A. S. (2013) Systematic review and meta-analysis on the work-related cause of de Quervain tenosynovitis: a critical appraisal of its recognition as an occupational disease. *Plastic and Reconstructive Surgery,* **132,** 1479–91.

Takala, E. P., Pehkonen, I., Forsman, M., Hansson, G. A., Mathiassen, S. E., Neumann, W. P., et al. (2010) Systematic evaluation of observational methods assessing biomechanical exposures at work. *Scandinavian Journal of Work and Environmental Health,* **36,** 3–24.

Trask, C., Mathiassen, S. E., Wahlstrom, J., and Forsman, M. (2014) Cost-efficient assessment of biomechanical exposure in occupational groups, exemplified by posture observation and inclinometry. *Scandinavian Journal of Work and Environmental Health,* **40,** 252–65.

Waddell, G. (2004) *The Back Pain Revolution.* Edinburgh: Churchill Livingstone.

Van Der Windt, D. A., Thomas, E., Pope, D. P., De Winter, A. F., MacFarlane, G. J., Bouter, L. M., and Silman, A. J. (2000) Occupational risk factors for shoulder pain: a systematic review. *Occupational and Environmental Medicine,* **57,** 433–42.

Van Dieen, J. H., Hoozemans, M. J., and Toussaint, H. M. (1999) Stoop or squat: a review of biomechanical studies on lifting technique. *Clinical Biomechanics (Bristol, Avon),* **14,** 685–96.

Verbeek, J. (2012) When work is related to disease, what establishes evidence for a causal relation? *Safety and Health at Work,* **3,** 110–16.

Verbeek, J., Martimo, K. P., Karppinen, J., Kuijer, P. P., Takala, E. P., and Viikari-Juntura, E. (2012) Manual material handling advice and assistive devices for preventing and treating back pain in workers: a Cochrane Systematic Review. *Occupational and Environmental Medicine,* **69,** 79–80.

Verhagen, A. P., Bierma-Zeinstra, S. M., Burdorf, A., Stynes, S. M., De Vet, H. C., and Koes, B. W. (2013) Conservative interventions for treating work-related complaints of the arm, neck or shoulder in adults. *Cochrane Database Systematic Review,* Cd008742.

Chapter 8

Lives lived longer: Chronic pain, subjective well-being, and occupation

Christopher Eccleston

Introduction

Populations worldwide are ageing. Lower rates of fertility and increased longevity are both contributing to the increase in the number of people aged 60 and older. The current estimate is that by 2030 this proportion of the population will rise from 10% to 22% (Bloom, 2011), equalling the adolescent population. The consequences of lives lived longer vary by geography, culture, public policy, and economics. However, it is clear that with greater longevity come greater morbidity and an increased need for long-term treatment or care. The subsequent macro-economic and policy changes present novel social and political challenges for which no one economy has yet been able to provide viable responses (Bloom et al., 2015).

For many, population changes are a cause for concern. Some see only spiralling social care costs, distorted pension and housing markets, and social problems caused largely by the weakening of savings, lower income-related tax recovery, and by disincentives to staying in the labour market for longer. There is fervent policy activity in discussing solutions to the perceived problem of a shrinking proportion of people in paid labour (e.g. Foster, 2018). For others, ageing populations and a life lived longer are cast as opportunities. For example, in their influential and well received treatise '100 year life', Gratton and Scott (2016) argue that if life expectancy projections remain unchanged, those born in 2010 can expect to live to 100, making our earlier benchmarking for later life of '60 and older' look outdated. They recognize that for some, especially those in mid-working life, it will be a challenge to alter long-held assumptions about the received three-part life order of training, working, and retirement. For others, however, the redesign of working lives could be liberatory. They argue that mixing these three components over a lifetime could produce new models welcomed by many. In a similar positive vein, Karl Pillemer has done much to reinvigorate the debate around positive ageing with his successful distillation of the legacy project. Through interview with many US 'seniors' he captured the wisdom of those who have lived full lives, documenting advice for everything from marriage and parenting, to how to avoid regret, and, of course, to how to understand working lives (Pillemer, 2012). At the centre of these discussions about longevity is a concern with the economic cost and contribution of an aging population, and perhaps less with the more abstract idea of social capital, in particular with the value of experience.

Social, economic, and personal assumptions about longevity, later life, and of work across the lifespan are all changing and changing radically. We are in flux. For those with pain, then, how far one is able, willing, or has the opportunity to work in later life, when the concepts of both 'work' and 'later life' are all in play provides even more challenge: almost a form of double jeopardy. In this chapter our focus is exactly on this problem. First, we start with a summary of the burden of pain in later life, and the current approach to prevention and treatment of chronic pain. Second, we then focus on the role of pain to alter one's subjective life course with an emphasis on identity, coping, and work re-engagement. Next, we summarize the evidence for pain management interventions and discuss the need for a contexualized approach to later life pain prevention, treatment, and emphasize the need for reform in both current and planned approaches. Finally, we end with the opportunities created by demographic changes, by workforce reform, and by communication technology, arguing for a radical change in our perspective of later life, later life employment, and the place of pain.

Pain in later life

Everyday pain, the type treated with distraction or with simple analgesics, does not appear to differ radically between countries. In a European study across eight major countries we found that in general the number of pain episodes reported each month did not differ across age groups, with a stable reported frequency of 1–2 episodes a month. The most notable age-related differences in the over-65 group were less knowledge about analgesics and belief in their efficacy, and greater worry about analgesic use (Vowles et al., 2014). The frequency of both pain and worry were elevated in Russia, a finding also reported in the Gallup World Poll in which 'countries of the former Soviet Union and eastern Europe' show almost twice the proportion of the 65–75-year-old population reporting 'pain yesterday' compared with those in 'high income English speaking countries' (Steptoe et al., 2015).

How far everyday pain is implicated in reduced quality of life or identified as a source of disability or distress is often missing from studies focused on only incidence or prevalence. A US study of an age-representative sample of 7601 older adults (65 years and older) focussed on how bothersome pain had been in the previous month, producing a prevalence of 52.9%, similar across the age bands, although slightly higher at 56% for the over 85s (Patel et al., 2013). This focus on pain that bothers gets us closer to what is important about pain. Although the prevalence of pain and how bothersome it is does not seem to change across the life span the stereotypical expectation of pain in later life as something to simply accept is common (Sarkisian, 2005). However, for some—and conservative estimates suggest this figure is 1 in 5 of adults—pain is chronic, i.e. having persisted for 3 months or longer and having become part of daily life (Breivik et al., 2006; Docking et al., 2011; van Hecke, 2014).

Chronic pain in later life, whether associated with cancer, disease of the musculoskeletal or somatosensory systems, or headache and migraine, is associated with increased mortality. In particular, severe chronic pain is associated with all-cause mortality and in particular circulatory system disease-related death (Torrance et al., 2010). Using a US sample and a different approach focusing on the probability of transition from any one pain-related state to another in later life, Zimmer and Rubin (2016) found that pain-free life expectancy is substantially reduced by an earlier experience of pain. In summarizing they state that: 'A 55-year-old male can expect 24.7 years of life, of which 17.3 are pain-free, 2.8 are with milder, and 4.5 are with severe pain. A similarly aged female has greater longevity—27.4 years—but extra years are lived with pain—3.1 with milder and 7.0 with severe pain. Thus, while the pain-free life expectancy of males and females across ages is about equal, females live more years with pain, and with more severe pain. As males and females age, life expectancy decreases. But, proportion of life expected with pain does not change.' (Zimmer and Rubin, 2016; p. 1174)[1]

For a minority, severe pain is a defining feature of later life and for most, intermittent episodes of pain are a frequent occurrence. Our focus in what follows is not on mortality, nor on context-free morbidity, but on the consequences of chronic pain, on disability, distress, and self-evaluation of subjective health and well-being. We know that the variation in subjective well-being, on pleasurable and meaningful experience, is affected by judgements of the effect of pain on a life lived as expected or as desired (Steptoe et al., 2015). Our approach is to focus on the meaning assigned in later life to goals still pursued or set aside, including goals thought of traditionally as occupational. We start with a developmental psychology view of normal ageing and the place pain can have in altering that normative trajectory.

Psychological ageing and later life

Psychological ageing is best thought of as social and cognitive development within context. Typically, that context is one defined by social expectations. One is normally allowed to be unskilled when young and expected to be wise when old. But each of us has a personal narrative of ageing and can, if called to account, tell our story of how we arrived 'here'. A useful model of ageing in the context of social and personal loss was provided by Brandtstädter and colleagues known as the dual processing model, and sometimes as the dual process model of coping. Their focus on coping is meant to capture the adjustment to goals that occur across life. This practical and pragmatic view of human psychology is unapologetically motivational. It assumes that we have, or can easily characterize, our motivations in terms of goals we are attempting to achieve. We recruit effort in the service of achieving those goals. The interest, however, is not in goal pursuit or achievement, but in what happens when those goals are frustrated (Brandtstädter and Renner, 1990; Brandtstädter and Rothermund, 2002).

When our goals are frustrated we have two broad responses. First we attempt to recruit further effort, remove social, physical, or personal barriers to success, and generally alter all external factors in order to achieve. This form of adaptation is known as 'assimilative'. Second, we can identify the goal as no longer reachable, maybe once

---

[1] Reproduced with permission from Zimmer Z. and Rubin S. (2016). Life expectancy with and without pain in the U.S. elderly population. *J Geontol A Biol Sci Med Sci.* 71(9): 1171–1176. https://doi.org/10.1093/gerona/glw028.

within reach when younger but now unrealistic. In this mode, we attempt to alter the meaning, relevance, and importance of the goal so that failure in reaching this goal is no longer frustrating. This form of adaptation is known as 'accommodative'. These two modes are not characterological; they are not personality types. These behavioural styles operate dynamically together. For a more concrete example, when should one stop trying to achieve a major competitive advantage in an elite sport. On failure one might assimilate to work harder, but after multiple and repeated failure one might accommodate and adapt one's goal as competitive advantage in an age-banded elite sport, or in an amateur sport. From this perspective, important are the choices to persist, how tenaciously to persist, when to disengage from an unachievable goal, and whether goal frustration produces lasting distress or adaptation in accommodating to a more achievable goal Ageing from this perspective is a dynamic process of assimilating and accommodating. Sometimes we need to pursue goals more avidly; sometimes we need to surrender them sooner. Normally that wisdom is gained in retrospect.

For many people this constant trade-off of motivation, goals, achievements, and adaptations occurs without observation. For some, there is discussion or self-reflection as a way to live one's life, although for many this process can become explicit at critical junctures such as job change, study, marriage, divorce, changing home, grief, illness, and incapacity. We are relatively resilient at coping with short-lived changes, including pain. Because pain functions to promote an awareness of potential harm, so the temporary suspension of goal pursuit and the adoption of a sick role is a normal and socially acceptable behaviour (Eccleston, 2016). It makes sense to withdraw from normal life and find something to take the pain away. However, when one has a chronic illness, one that is not going away, then aging well becomes a significant challenge. Life can be set on a different course, including one's relationship with work or occupation. In 2016, we outlined the three major challenges to ageing caused by chronic pain, narrated in terms of their ability to threaten core psychological components: identity, depression, and disability (Eccleston et al., 2016).

The challenge of chronic pain to ageing well

Identity is the least examined but probably the most critical of the three challenges. Identity challenge is a major theme emerging from qualitative research: when asked patients will report that pain challenges one's core sense of who one is, normally narrated as an unwelcome loss (Harris et al., 2003). Beyond role loss, pain can distort identity (Vlaeyen et al., 2016). That distortion can extend and become far reaching (Morley et al., 2005). For some people, one's identity can be enmeshed so closely with pain that it becomes difficult to think of any aspect of one's life as being free of pain, including one's idea about any future. Being able to think about oneself as separate from pain can be difficult, fraught with uncertainty. What used to be considered important, i.e. work or professional life, can become unimportant. For some, a job is a means to maintain an identity as a provider. When family is everything, work is a practical means of support, and the identity of breadwinner is critical (Williams, 2017). For others, work is as much a means of practical support as a core part of identity. To lose a professional identity earlier because of pain can be experienced as a catastrophic loss not only of current self, but of a future desired self (Morley and Eccleston, 2004). At end of life, Brandtstädter and colleagues argue that one reaches almost an ultimate accommodation in liberating one from the dominance of self-concern, in what they call a final decentration (Brandtstädter et al., 2010).

Depression is a constant companion of many people with chronic pain and can be a feature of later life pain. Untreated or poorly managed pain is a risk factor for later life pain (Calvó-Perxas et al., 2016), more for men than women. Depression is often a compound noun for a range of related distressing symptoms, including failure in motivation, loneliness, and anger. There is little research on the protective factors on the development of mental health problems by people with chronic pain in later life, but there is some evidence that cognitive function and social support are critical. Maintaining complex cognitive tasks and delivering them in a social context protects not from pain but from depression in pain (Lee et al., 2016). Accommodating to the losses of chronic pain can fuel long-term depression, creating social isolation and diminished opportunity for activity. People in later life are often encouraged to accept pain and the losses associated with it. Many people, however, find the concept of acceptance too difficult as it requires a fundamental shift in belief; for many it is a pejorative term (Risdon et al., 2003). That said, there is preliminary evidence that some older patients are more receptive to the idea of accommodating to pain than younger patients who might put more effort into assimilative coping (Wetherell et al., 2016).

Loss of role, physical function, and physical activity combine in disability to produce a range of mobility and independence changes. The change can be sudden or gradual. Reductions in physical function in general predict later reductions of physical activity (Metti et al., 2018), but when physical activity is painful then functional loss is exacerbated. Fear of movement and the consequences of harm can translate into habits of avoidance that lead in turn to altered gait, fear of falling, and more pain. Occupation in this context can become the first casualty. Uncertainty over future functional abilities, fear of dependency, and dominant cultural stereotypes of ageing can significantly confuse what might be possible with pain in later life (Morden et al., 2017). Accommodative coping as the relinquishing of an unachievable goal and the adoption of new goals can be fear and depression masquerading as acceptance. These decisions are made more difficult by daily variations in the subjective judgement of ageing caused by current demands (Kotter-Grün et al., 2015). This assimilation–accommodation tension has been called the major task of aging: when to adjust and when to endure (Eckerblad et al., 2015). The extent to which a narrowing life is an inevitably unwelcome aspect of ageing is unclear.

In Box 8.1 and 8.2 we give two illustrative examples of people facing normal ageing interrupted by pain with a focus on work and occupation. In the first example (Box 8.1), Kevin exemplifies the push–pull dilemma of knowing when to adjust and when to endure, operating in an environment of unwelcome acceptance of a sudden loss of role. In the second example (Box 8.2), Mavis exemplifies a successful shifting between roles adopting a later life occupation blended with ever-present caring responsibilities. In both, 'work' and its effect in buffering identity maintenance and positive self-regard, is a prominent feature.

Box 8.1 Early retirement for reasons of ill-health

Kevin is 63 years old, a builder who works on construction sites. He has had periods of management responsibility, managing logistics, sites, and people, but later in his career chose to go back to the construction site stating that he ' … does not enjoy management, likes the camaraderie of work, enjoys being outside, and especially enjoys seeing the immediate rewards of his labour'.

Kevin has repeated episodes of back pain and the last had him off work for 6 months. He is going through a process of early retirement on illness grounds. He has become exhausted and frustrated at attempting to find a cure for his pain, attempting to alter his work pattern, and persuade his employees to alter the work demands. Those around him see his departure as 'early retirement'; he experiences it as a major loss as he had expected to work until past 70 years. He judges that he has valuable skills and experience that he still wants to use but feels ' … rejected, ignored, and passed over'.

Eventually the anger, social stigma of being in pain, and the repeated attempts to assimilate (change the world) to keep him at work leave him depressed and over-whelmed by loss and fear of future loss. 'Retirement … ' [he says] ' … feels like a concept from another generation, from another time. I like to work and I am being denied the opportunity by pain and people's acceptance that it is ok for me to retire because I am in my 60s.' He is moving toward accommodation (trying to adapt his goals) but this is a major challenge for him. Other people talk to him about needing to 'accept' his position, but he experiences this as giving up, as a 'surrender'.

For Kevin, the problem of chronic pain is tied closely to his identity. The loss is of current and future self, the stigma of becoming a person 'retired due to ill health' and the uncertainty of future occupation and identity are highly threatening. Accommodation may occur naturally, or may not. It could be supported thera-peutically or with social support if such services were available.

Pain management in later life

Pain in later life is typically complex, complicated so often by multimorbidity. The challenge of chronic pain management is to provide a tailored therapy in the context of obesity, arthritis, diabetes, depression, cancer, and by frailty. Pharmacological ap-proaches are a common mainstay of treatment (Reid et al., 2015), but the evidence is undermined largely by the absence of older people and patients with complex pres-entations in primary clinical trials of analgesic medications. The optimal treatment approach is to provide a multidisciplinary and multimodal programme including later-life medicine, social work, psychology, and family members. The reality, however, of later life pain management is that the role falls largely to primary care providers, who may feel unskilled (Mills et al., 2016). Further, many people in later life live in organized residential facilities which pose a specific challenge to optimal pain care,

Box 8.2 Retirement means 'checking out'

Mavis is 78 years old. She has had many paid jobs in her life, from working in a munitions factory to working as a nursing auxiliary, working in customer facing roles, and in later life running a busy architect's office. Additionally, she has always had caring responsibilities. She lost a child from leukaemia when she was 36, a husband from a stroke when she was 60, and nursed her own mother at home until she died when Mavis was 73. She has two further children and five grandchildren who live locally and she frequently cares for. She has suffered trigeminal neuralgia for 30 years describing it as her 'demon', an ever-present reminder of her limits.

Family and caring for family is her core motivation and she values being able to be helpful and supportive very highly. Over her life her goals have constantly changed but have always been in the service of her values. She describes her chronic pain as at its most debilitating when it stops her from ' ... being who she wants to be, being useful and being a full part of her family.' When the pain started she pursued many possible treatments, but eventually decided that the pain was 'here to stay' and she needed to adjust what she could do with the pain.

The idea of a 100-year life is not revolutionary to Mavis. She considers it a male idea. Women have always been operating in multiple roles (earning, caring, providing) and jobs have always been temporary or likely to end at some point. Life has been a series of multiple engagements driven by the need to provide and a need to feel useful. For Mavis she realized that the pain she was experiencing started to dominate her life, and the search for a cure was having more widespread devastating effects on her as a person. Attempts at assimilation were starting to interfere. Her accommodation emerges slowly as she found her new limits. Accommodating to pain brings new challenges. Mostly they are social and interpersonal. Mavis learned early on that although she adjusted to having pain as part of her life, people around her found it hard to understand. Talk about pain provokes talk about action: 'you should get that sorted'; 'you should not have to suffer'. And close behind talk about action is an implication of irresponsibility: ' ... why are you choosing to suffer?'

For Mavis, chronic pain is another adjustment, another change, another job to do. She characterizes her life as one of constant challenge and change. The losses she has had have changed her identity, and the pain she has fundamentally changes her. But her life has been one of ageing through short-term assimilation and longer-term accommodation. For her, those accommodations have strengthened her and allowed her to stay working. For Mavis working is best defined as contributing through caring. Retirement does not make sense in her world, and will mean 'checking out' when one leaves the world altogether, when she dies.

especially where there are common communication problems which make the appropriate assessment of pain difficult, and under-treatment common (Tan et al., 2015).

Psychological approaches to helping people adjust to pain in later life are developing. The traditional approach, using cognitive behavioural therapy (CBT), has been to focus on psychological barriers to change. Often CBT is offered within a rehabilitation context which promotes a return to function (Williams et al., 2012). In our language CBT aims to reduce the significance of the interruption (making it less threatening), reduce the interference in returning people to function, and reduce any distortion in identity caused by pain. Later life, however, is a different context. First, assimilation is not always fruitless. Although many patients have had pain for many years, an assessment of what can be changed in the environment may never have been undertaken. A pharmacological review, occupational therapy, and physiotherapy assessment could be more important in altering barriers to function than any psychological approach. Occupational therapy, in particular, with a focus on valued and personally relevant roles, is essential. Second, and perhaps only after such an assessment, accommodation focused on an uncoupling from unachievable goals to an adoption of new goals within the same value-frame, needs to be considered within the context of later life development and growth.

Karl Pillemer describes beautifully the richness and depth of later life occupation, and in particular the active reconstruction of remembered events into guidance on how to age wisely (Pillemer, 2012). The dominant stereotypes of ageing in many cultures lead to a view of people in later life being occupationally passive. The opposite is often true. People are often working hard on roles that can be invisible, not fitting the dominant view of labour, but can have a major effect of workforce participation overall. For example, grandparent care in the UK has been estimated to increase mothers' involvement in paid work by 33% (Kanji, 2018). Pain in this complex interrelated context has the possibility of affecting not only the individual's occupational participation but also the participation of other adults.

Opportunities in later life pain management

Given that many countries have ageing populations, characterized by a larger number of people entering later life with co-morbidities, many of which are associated with pain (Eccleston et al., 2018), it is clear that the current pain management workforce is inadequate to meet current and future need. There are too few individuals with appropriate expertise, no workforce planning, and no training or development. Such a widespread absence in planning for a major population change is an opportunity for novel development. There are three areas of immediate opportunity.

First, we propose a radical rethinking of the delivery of self-management interventions. The case studies show the complexity of individual presentations and the danger in assuming common goals. Occupation, broadly understood, is important for people in later life, but the return to a previous occupation is not always desirable, desired, or possible. Accommodating to new occupation often requires comprehensive assessment of how new roles might be considered, experimented with, and adopted. Further, understanding the relational context of later life occupation is likely to be important.

Many people are actively engaged in social and caring structures in provision as well as receipt of care. A modern CBT tailored for people in later life living with chronic pain needs to be socially and contextually relevant.

Second, there are opportunities for the more widespread use of information technology in the assessment of interruption, interference, and identity disruption. In a recent project, we ran a consensus conference to determine the research agenda in mobile health innovation and later life pain (Wetherington et al., 2018). The priorities for research focused on the need to increase the uptake and accessibility of existing and future technologies for older users, to ensure that a holistic approach to pain management was taken, and to research the integration of sensor technology in any resultant product or service. In addition, there was a recognition of the importance of working in concert with industrial and commercial developers, not only with university, health, or third sector partners. Commercial providers of technological solutions in long-term conditions need to ensure that later life experience is fully accounted for. User involvement in the design of solutions was key, in particular to counter the stereotype of people being fearful of technology. Paradoxically, there was also a warning that too strong a reliance on technology to allow communication at a distance could inadvertently increase isolation and loneliness. From a commercial perspective, there was a need to identify more clearly the 'later life' care market which is currently difficult to quantify, but goes beyond the focus on disposable income, or the so called 'grey dollar'.

Third, there is a major opportunity to totally redesign how we think about later life, and so later life pain, which spreads across domains, from social policy to economic planning, from technology design to service development, and in social medicine and education. There is an active discussion on the intergenerational transmission of expectations of pain and analgesia, typically from parents to children, with different views on the importance of parents' own experience and their expression of pain is in explaining child pain and behaviour (Higgins et al., 2015). Much of this literature is concerned with younger children. One study of parents with pain and its effects on adult children showed that adult children are not affected by parental pain in the same way (Pillemer et al., 2017). There are no studies I could find on the backward transmission of pain from a younger to an older person. Social innovation is necessary in bridging the gap between generations in pain and analgesic beliefs and expectations, and in novel interventions in intergenerational communication for positive benefits in promoting effective coping and living well with chronic pain.

Conclusion

With ageing populations and the rise in longevity, working lives are changing and extending. The opportunities for pain to interrupt, interfere, and alter working identities has increased. People in later life are already working in multiple roles, are active in switching between roles, and offer experience and wisdom on pain management that could be shared more widely. For some, however, chronic pain can detrimentally alter natural ageing and halt personal development. Critical to this is the subjective judgement of who one is, how to manage the interruption from pain, and how much interference in life is inevitable and unchangeable. Many people cope with the changes of pain without professional help and others seek support. Although the current approaches to helping people learn to self-manage chronic pain, and recovery from the identity assault of pain are in their infancy, the early steps are promising. However, there are significant opportunities in both social and technological development that could be used to innovate new solutions and novel ways to live intergenerationally with pain.

References

Bloom, D. E. (2011) 7 billion and counting. *Science*, **333**, 562–9.

Bloom, D. E., Chatterji, S., Kowal, P., Lloyd-Sherlock, P., McKee, M., Rechel, B., et al. (2015) Macroeconomic implications of population ageing and selected policy responses. *Lancet*, **385**, 649–57.

Brandtstädter, J., and Renner, G. (1990) Tenacious goal pursuit and flexible goal adjustment: explication and age-related analysis of assimilative and accommodative strategies of coping. *Psychology and Aging*, **5**, 58–67.

Brandtstädter, J., and Rothermund, K. (2002) The life-course dynamics of goal pursuit and goal adjustment: a two process framework. *Developmental Review*, **22**, 117–50.

Brandtstädter, J., Rothermund, K., Kranz, D., and Kühn, W. (2010) Final decentrations: personal goals, rationality perspectives, and the awareness of life's finitude. *European Psychologist*, **15**, 152–63.

Breivik, H., Collett, B., Ventafridda, V., Cohen, R, and Gallacher, D. (2006) Survey of chronic pain in Europe: prevalence, impact on daily life, and treatment. *European Journal of Pain*, **10**, 287–333.

Calvó-Perxa, L., Vilalta-Franch, J., Turró-Garrig, O., López-Pousa, S., and Garre-Olmo J. (2016) Gender differences in depression and pain: A two year follow-up study of the Survey of Health, Ageing and Retirement in Europe. *Journal of Affective Disorders*, **193**, 157–64.

Docking, R. E., Fleming, J., Brayne, C., Zhao, J, McFarlane, G. J., and Jones, G.T. (2011) Epidemiology of back pain in older adults: prevalence and risk factors for back pain onset. *Rheumatology*, **50**, 1645–53.

Eccleston, C. (2016) *Embodied: the Psychology of Physical Sensation.* Oxford: Oxford University Press.

Eccleston, C., Wells, C., and Morlion, B. (eds). (2018) *European Pain Management.* Oxford: Oxford University Press.

Eccleston, C., Tabor, A., Edwards, R. T., and Keogh E. (2016) Psychological approaches to coping with pain in later life. *Clinical and Geriatric Medicine*, **32**, 763–71.

Eckerblad, J., Theander, K., Ekdahl, A., Jaarsma, T., and Hellstrom I. (2015) To adjust and endure: a qualitative study of symptom burden in older people with multimorbidity. *Applied Nursing Research*, **28**, 322–7.

Foster, L. Active ageing, pensions and retirement in the UK. (2018) *Journal of Population Ageing*, **11**, 117–32.

Gratton, L., and Scott, A. (2016) *The 100-year Life. Living and Working in an Age of Longevity.* London: Bloomsbury.

Harris, S., Morley, S., and Barton, S. B. (2003) Role loss and emotional adjustment in chronic pain. *Pain*, **105**, 363–70.

Higgins, K. S., Birnie, K. A., Chambers, C. T., Wilson, A. C., Caes, L., Clark, A. J., et al. (2015) Offspring of parents with chronic pain: a systematic review and meta-analysis of pain, health, psychological, and family outcomes. *Pain*, **156**, 2256–66.

Kanji, S. (2018) Grandparent are: A key factor in mothers' labour force participation in the UK. *Journal of Social Policy*, **47**, 523–42.

Kotter-Grün, D., Neupert, S. D., and Stephan, Y. (2015) Feeling old today? Daily health, stressors, and affect explain day-to-day variability in subjective age. *Psychology and Health*, **30**, 1470–85.

Lee, J. E., Kahana, B., and Kahana, E. (2016) Social support and cognitive functioning as resources for elderly persons with chronic arthritis pain. *Aging and Mental Health*, **20**, 370–9.

Metti, A. L., Best, J. R., Shaaban, C. E., Ganguli, M., and Rosano, C. (2018) Longitudinal changes in physical function and physical activity in older adults. *Age and Ageing*, **47**, 558–64.

Mills, S., Torrance, N., and Smith, B. H. (2016) Identification and management of chronic pain in primary care: a review. *Current Psychiatry Reports* **18**, 22.

Morden, A., Jinks, C., and Ong, B. N. (2017) Temporally divergent significant meanings, biographical disruption and self-management for chronic joint pain. *Health*, **21**, 357–74.

Morley, S., Davies, C., and Barton S. (2005) Possible selves in chronic pain: self-pain enmeshment, adjustment and acceptance. *Pain*, **115**, 84–94.

Morley, S., and Eccleston, C. (2004) The object of fear in pain. In: Asmundson, G. J. G., Valeyen, J. W. S., and Crombez, G. (eds.) *Understanding and Treating the Fear of Pain*. Oxford: Oxford University Press, 163–88.

Patel, K. V., Guralnik, J. M., Dansie, E. J., and Turk, D. C. (2013) Prevalence and impact of pain among older adults in the United States: findings from the 2011 National Health and Aging Trends Study. *Pain*, **154**, 2649–57.

Pillemer, K. (2012) *30 Lessons for Living. Tried and True Advice from the Wisest Americans*. New York: Penguin.

Pillemer, K., Riffin, C., Suitor, J. J., Peng, S., and Reid, M. C. (2017) The impact of older parents' pain symptoms on adult children. *Pain Medicine*, **12**, 2316–24.

Reid, M. C., Eccleston, C., and Pillemer, K. (2015) Chronic pain in older adults. *BMJ*, **350**, h532.

Risdon, A., Eccleston, C., Crombez, G., and McCracken L. (2003) How can we learn to live with pain? A Q-methodological analysis of the diverse understandings of acceptance of chronic pain. *Social Science and Medicine*, **56**, 375–86.

Sarkisian, C. A., Steers, N., Hays, R. D., and Mangione, C. M. (2005) Development of the 12-item expectations regarding aging survey. *Gerontologist*, **45**, 240–8.

Steptoe, A., Deaton, A., and Stone, A. A. (2015) Subjective wellbeing, health, and ageing. *Lancet*, **385**, 640–8.

Tan, E. C. K., Jokanovic, N., Koponen, M. P. H., Thomas, D., Hilmer, S. N., and Bell, J. S. (2015) Prevalence of analgesic use and pain in people with and without dementia or cognitive impairment in aged care facilities: A systematic review and meta-analysis. *Current Clinical Pharmacology*, **10**, 194–203.

Torrance, N., Elliott, A. M., Lee, A. J., and Smith, B. H. (2010) Severe chronic pain is associated with increased 10 year mortality. A cohort record linkage study. *European Journal of Pain*, **14**, 380–6.

van Hecke, O., Austin, S. K., Khan, R. A., Smith, B. H., Torrance, N. (2014) Neuropathic pain in the general population: a systematic review of epidemiological studies. *Pain*, **155**, 654–62.

Vlaeyen, J. W. S., **Morley, S.,** and **Crombez, G.** (2016) The experimental analysis of the interruptive, interfering and identity-distorting effects of chronic pain. *Behaviour Research and Therapy*, **86**, 23–34.

Vowles, K. E., **Rosser, B., Januszewicz, P., Morlion, B., Evers, S.,** and **Eccleston,** C. (2014) Everyday pain, analgesic beliefs, and analgesic behaviours in Europe and Russia: An epidemiological survey and analysis. *European Journal of Hospital Pharmacy*, **21**, 39–44.

Wetherell, J. L., **Petkus, A. J., Alonso-Fernandez, M., Bower, E. S., Steiner, A. R. W.,** and **Afari,** N. (2016) Age moderates response to acceptance and commitment therapy vs. cognitive behavioral therapy for chronic pain. *International Journal of Geriatric Psychiatry*, **31**, 302–8.

Wetherington, E., **Eccleston, C., Gay, G., Gooberman-Hill, R., Schofield, P., Bacon, E.,** et al. (2018) Establishing a research agenda on mobile health technologies and later-life pain using an evidence-based consensus conference approach. *Clinical Journal of Pain*, **12**, 1416–23.

Williams, A.C. de C., **Eccleston, C.,** and **Morley, S.** (2012) Psychological therapies for the management of chronic pain (excluding headache) in adults. *Cochrane Database of Systematic Reviews*, Issue 11. Art. No.: CD007407. DOI: 10.1002/14651858.CD007407.pub3.

Williams, J.C. (2017) *White Working Class: Overcoming Class Cluelessness in America.* Boston: Harvard Business Review Press.

Zimmer, Z., and **Rubin,** S. (2016) Life expectancy with and without pain in the U.S. elderly population. *Journals of Gerontology. Series A, Biological Sciences and Medical Sciences*, **71**, 1171–6.

Section 3

Interventions

Chapter 9

The psychology of pain-related disability: Implications for intervention

Michael J. L. Sullivan, Stephania Donayre Pimentel, and Catherine Paré

Introduction

Musculoskeletal disorders are considered one of the leading causes of disability. In North America, musculoskeletal disorders are the most expensive non-malignant health condition affecting the working-age population (Crook et al., 2002). The prevalence of pain-related disability associated with musculoskeletal disorders has been increasing steadily in spite of numerous policy, prevention, and intervention initiatives launched to date (Overaas et al., 2017).

Considerable research has been conducted on trajectories of recovery following musculoskeletal injury. Although approximately 50% of individuals who sustain a work-disabling musculoskeletal injury return to work within 4 weeks, a significant proportion of individuals remain work-disabled for prolonged periods of time (da Silva et al., 2017). Individuals who remain work-disabled at 3-months post-injury have a high likelihood of permanent disability (da Silva et al., 2017).

One of the challenges in this area of research has been to discern the variables that distinguish between individuals who will recover following injury and those who will remain occupationally disabled. Initial research in this area focused primarily on symptom severity and injury characteristics as possible risk factors of prolonged pain and disability (Lanier and Stockton, 1988). The failure to identify reliable medical or physical predictors of prolonged work disability prompted consideration of the non-medical variables that might be influencing return-to-work outcomes following musculoskeletal injury (Verkerk et al., 2012).

Over the past two decades, investigators have expanded the search for determinants of prolonged pain and disability to include psychological, behavioural, and social variables (Turk and Okifuji, 2002). There has been particular interest in identifying modifiable risk factors for persistent pain and disability (Sullivan et al., 2005). The identification of modifiable risk factors could lay the foundation for risk-targeted interventions that might prevent the development of pain-related disability following injury.

This chapter examines what is currently known about psychological risk factors for problematic recovery following musculoskeletal injury. The review is selective as opposed to exhaustive, with emphasis on variables and interventions that have been systematically evaluated. The present focus on psychological risk factors for pain-related disability should not be construed as a neglect of other possible contributors to work-disability. It is recognized that there are many other risk factors (e.g. biomedical, physical, environmental) that influence recovery and rehabilitation outcomes following injury.

Pain-related psychological risk factors

Twenty years ago, heated debates would arise during discussions about the influence of psychological factors in the development and maintenance of disability. Today there is little room for debate. Indeed, research has been consistent in showing that certain psychosocial variables can increase the risk for pronounced and prolonged disability following musculoskeletal injury (Leeuw et al., 2007; Pincus et al., 2002; Sullivan, 2003; Sullivan et al., 2005). Five psychological cognitive variables have emerged as consistent and robust predictors of disability across a wide range of debilitating health and mental health conditions. These are recovery expectancies, self-efficacy, pain catastrophizing, perceived injustice, and health beliefs (Sullivan et al., 2011; Edwards et al., 2016). Comorbid mental health problems, such as depression and post-traumatic stress disorder, have also been shown to impede recovery and return to work following musculoskeletal injury. A brief summary of the evidence on the relation between pain-related psychosocial risk factors and work-disability following musculoskeletal injury is provided below.

Psychological risk factors—cognitive variables

Recovery expectancies

Recovery expectancies have emerged as one of the strongest psychological predictors of prolonged work disability following musculoskeletal injury. Recovery expectancies have been broadly defined as a person's prediction of the likelihood of recovery (or return to work) following injury. Findings have been consistent in showing that less positive, or more negative, recovery expectancies are strong predictors of who will return to work following a debilitating musculoskeletal injury and who will remain work-disabled (Carriere et al., 2015).

The operational definition of recovery expectancies has varied considerably across studies. In some studies, injured individuals have been asked about their expected duration of sick leave, their perceived risk of not recovering, the likelihood of returning to work within a particular time period, or the probability of returning to work without restriction (Iles et al., 2008). In spite of variations in the operational definitions, findings have been consistent in showing that recovery expectancies are important prognostic indicators of return to work outcomes (Carriere et al., 2015; Carroll et al., 2016; Iles et al., 2012).

Several investigations have examined the prospective association between recovery expectancies and return to work outcomes in individuals suffering from a wide range of musculoskeletal conditions. Cole et al. (2002) reported that injured workers' expectations of slower recovery were consistently associated with longer duration of time loss claims. Du Bois and Donceel (2008) reported that work-disabled individuals who were less than 100% certain that they would return to work within the next 6 months were four times less likely to return to work during that time period. Turner et al. (2006) showed that injured workers who reported 'low certainty' of return to work within the next 6 months had over 12 times the number of disability days than those who were 'extremely certain' of returning to work. Hallegraeff et al. (2012) examined the relationship between low expectancies and work disability across ten studies of individuals with low back pain. Results revealed that individuals with low recovery expectancies were more than twice as likely to be work-disabled than those with high recovery expectancies 3 months or more following the onset of pain.

There are indications that recovery expectancies might be one of the vehicles through which other pain-related psychological risk factors exert their influence on return to work outcomes. In a sample of work-disabled individuals with whiplash injuries, Carriere et al. (2015) showed that recovery expectancies fully mediated the relation between fear of re-injury and prolonged work-disability. Research suggests that the relation between pain catastrophizing, perceived injustice, depression, and work-disability might also be partially or fully mediated by recovery expectancies (Carriere, Thibault, and Sullivan, 2015a; Carriere et al., 2015b; Carriere et al., 2017).

Research and theory suggest that outcome expectancies might represent the final common pathway of a variety of psychological influences on behaviour (Bandura, 1977; Carriere et al., 2015a; Kirsch, 1985). Bandura has suggested that expectancies impact behaviour by interfering with the investment of effort and motivation required to achieve an outcome (Bandura, 1977). Low expectancies might also diminish an individual's persistence or efforts towards goal pursuits (Lackner et al., 1996). In individuals with musculoskeletal injuries, negative expectancies might lead to reduced motivation for participating in rehabilitation interventions. Low motivation consequent to negative expectancies could also take the form of non-compliance, non-adherence, or missed appointments for treatments intended to promote recovery. In addition, clients' verbalizations of negative expectancies might have a negative impact on the quality of the working alliance with the treating clinician.

Little is currently known about how negative recovery expectancies develop. It is possible that communication from health-care professionals might play a significant role in the development in individuals' recovery expectancies. Medical professionals who voice their opinions about a patient's inability to resume occupational tasks might inadvertently be setting in motion the conditions for a self-fulfilling prophecy. It is also possible that information obtained through media, internet, or significant others might play a role in the development of negative recovery expectancies. There are indications that individual difference variables such as catastrophizing or optimism might also influence recovery expectancies (Peters et al., 2007).

Self-efficacy

Self-efficacy was originally defined as 'beliefs in one's capabilities to organize and execute the course of action required to produce given attainments' (Bandura, 1977). Self-efficacy is a particular form of expectancy, as it is a probabilistic judgment about the future occurrence of a specific outcome. Bandura (1977) distinguished between two forms of expectancies related to behavioural outcomes: outcome expectancies and efficacy expectancies. Outcome expectancies refer to individuals' estimates that a given behaviour will result in a given outcome. Efficacy expectancies refer to the confidence individuals have that they possess the ability to successfully execute the behaviour required to yield a given outcome. Under conditions where individuals possess the necessary skills for execution of a particular behaviour, and when adequate incentives are in place, efficacy expectancies are said to be a major determinant of individuals' activity choices, and the effort they will expend to attain desired outcomes (Bandura, 1977).

In pain research, self-efficacy has been operationally defined in terms of one's overall confidence in the ability to deal with symptoms, stresses, or limitations associated with a pain condition, or in terms of the ability to manage, control, or decrease specific components of symptoms or disability (e.g. ability to decrease pain or complete certain activities in spite of pain) (Nicholas, 2007). Self-efficacy judgments are considered to be most predictive of proximal behaviour (Bandura, 1977). A measure of functional self-efficacy was developed by Barry et al. (2003). On this scale, respondents are asked to rate their confidence in their ability to carry out ten different activities of daily living. More recently, Brouwer et al. (2015) developed a scale to assess individuals' self-efficacy specific to the challenges of resuming occupational activities.

Several studies have reported that high levels of self-efficacy are associated with shorter periods of work-disability in individuals with musculoskeletal conditions (Lackner et al., 1996; Sarda et al., 2009). In a 10-month follow-up study, Brouwer et al. (2011) found a significant association between self- efficacy and the time to return to work in work-disabled individuals receiving treatment for a musculoskeletal condition. A 2-year prospective study examined the association between self-efficacy and return to work outcomes in individuals who had sustained musculoskeletal injuries (Richard et al., 2011). Higher scores on a measure of self-efficacy prospectively predicted successful return to work. Dionne et al. (2006) examined predictors of work absence in a sample of over 1000 individuals receiving primary care for disabling back pain. High levels of self-efficacy at initial assessment predicted fewer days of work absence over the next 2 years.

According to Bandura (1977), self-efficacy expectancies develop as a result of a number of experiential and social learning factors. Past experience with success or failure in producing specific outcomes are posited to influence individuals' confidence to produce such outcomes in the future. Vicarious experience, exposure to information, and the attributions made for outcomes are also considered to influence the development of self-efficacy expectancies (Bandura, 1977).

Pain catastrophizing

Pain catastrophizing has been identified as a key prognostic variable for prolonged work disability following musculoskeletal injury. Pain catastrophizing has been broadly defined as an 'exaggerated negative orientation to actual or anticipated pain comprising elements of rumination, magnification and helplessness' (Sullivan et al., 2001). Over 1000 studies have documented a relation between pain catastrophizing and adverse pain outcomes (Sullivan et al., 2001; Quartana et al., 2009). Pain catastrophizing has been associated with pain severity and pain-related disability in patients with musculoskeletal pain, even when controlling for medical status variables (Sullivan et al., 2001; Sullivan et al., 2005).

A relation between pain catastrophizing and work-disability was first reported by Burton and colleagues in 1995. In a prospective survey of patients seeking primary care for low back pain, high scores on a measure of pain catastrophizing were almost seven times more predictive of long-term disability than clinical or historical variables (Burton et al., 1995). Several subsequent investigations also supported a relation between scores on measures of catastrophizing and longer periods of sick-leave and work disability (Sullivan et al., 2005). Numerous correlational and prospective studies have shown that high levels of catastrophizing in individuals with musculoskeletal injuries are associated with more severe disability and prolonged work absence (Gauthier et al., 2006; Sullivan et al., 1998; Sullivan et al., 2005). In many studies, pain catastrophizing has been shown to contribute unique variance to the prediction of return to work outcomes, even when controlling for other disability-relevant variables such as pain severity, fear of re-injury, or depression (Sullivan et al., 2005; Carriere et al., 2015a).

Research has begun to explore the pathways through which pain catastrophizing might exert its negative impact on recovery trajectories. Pain catastrophizing has been shown to be associated with disability-relevant variables such as heightened display of pain behaviours (Thibault et al., 2008), increased analgesic intake (Jacobsen and Butler, 1996), prolonged bed rest following injury (Verbunt et al., 2008), depression (Sullivan et al., 2006), and dysfunctional pain modulation (Goodin et al., 2009). Pain catastrophizing has also been shown to be associated with poor response to a range of pain management interventions. For example, high scores on pain catastrophizing have been associated with less pain reduction following joint injection (Smith et al., 2013), radiofrequency neurotomy (Smith et al., 2016), and multidisciplinary rehabilitation (Scott et al., 2014). Pain catastrophizing has been shown to predict poor response to physical therapy (Bergbom et al., 2011), analgesic medication (Mankovsky et al., 2012), and surgical interventions (Pavlin et al., 2005).

The emerging body of research suggests that pain catastrophizing might adversely affect occupational re-engagement by contributing to ongoing pain, either through its effects on endogenous pain modulation or by attenuating treatment response. Pain catastrophizing might also trigger a cascade of cognitive, emotional, and behavioural responses that further complicate recovery and add to the burden of disability.

The origins of pain catastrophizing have been addressed primarily from a social learning perspective. It has been suggested that, as a function of a learning history characterized by heightened pain experience, catastrophizers may develop 'pain schema' about the high threat value of painful stimuli and about their inability to effectively manage the stress associated with painful experiences (Sullivan et al., 2001). Once activated, these pain schemas might influence emotional or cognitive functioning in a manner that leads to heightened pain experience. A recent study, however, points to the potential heritability of pain catastrophizing. In a large twin study, Trost et al. (2015) reported findings suggesting there was a genetic basis for pain catastrophizing. The heritability of pain catastrophizing might account for its overlap with indices of pathophysiological pain processing and its resistance to change through intervention (Quartana et al., 2009; Schutze et al., 2018).

Perceived injustice

Clinical anecdotes abound of persistent pain sufferers who feel they have been victimized either as a direct result of their injury or indirectly by injury-related sequelae (Aceves-Avila et al., 2004; McParland et al., 2011). An internet search quickly reveals numerous attestations that emphasize the injustice of living with pain: 'What did I do to deserve this?', 'I wish he could see what he has done to my life', and, 'Nothing will ever make up for what I have gone through.' Such attestations reflect at once elements of the magnitude of loss, the irreparability of loss, and a sense of unfairness (McParland and Whyte 2008; Sullivan et al., 2008).

DeGood and Kiernan (1996) provided one of the first empirical reports on the negative consequences of perceived injustice in individuals with pain conditions. In this study, individuals with chronic pain who blamed their employer for their injury, compared to those who did not blame an external source, reported significantly more emotional distress, expected less benefit from treatment, and were more likely to indicate that previous treatment had worsened their condition. The authors suggested that the efforts devoted to finding and ascribing blame for one's injury might detract from the investment of cognitive and emotional resources required to benefit fully from treatment. Since the early work of DeGood and Kiernan, perceived injustice has emerged as a powerful psychological predictor of delayed recovery following injury (Sullivan et al., 2008).

In the context of debilitating injury, perceived injustice has been conceptualized as an appraisal process characterized by a tendency to construe one's losses as severe and irreparable, and to attribute blame to others for one' suffering (Sullivan et al., 2008). In a prospective study of individuals with musculoskeletal injuries, Sullivan et al. (2008) reported that high scores on a measure of perceived injustice predicted work-disability at 1-year follow-up, even when controlling for initial pain severity, catastrophizing, depression, and pain-related fears. This was an important study in that it highlighted that perceived injustice was not simply a variant of other known psychosocial risk factors, but rather had unique predictive value over and above that afforded by other known psychosocial risk factors, such as catastrophizing, depression, or fear. The results of two subsequent prospective studies showed that high scores on the Injustice Experiences Questionnaire (IEQ), at the time of admission to a rehabilitation programme, were associated with longer periods of work disability following musculoskeletal injury (Scott and Sullivan 2012; Scott et al., 2013).

Perceived injustice has also been associated with delayed recovery of mental health problems consequent to musculoskeletal injury. Sullivan et al. (2009) examined the predictors of recovery from post-traumatic stress symptoms in a sample of individuals with recent onset cervical sprain injuries who were participating in a multidisciplinary rehabilitation programme. Individuals who scored high on a measure of perceived injustice were less likely to show recovery from their post-traumatic stress symptoms than individuals with low scores on perceived injustice. High scores on perceived injustice have also been shown to interfere with recovery of depressive symptoms in individuals who have sustained musculoskeletal injuries (Scott et al., 2015).

To date, the relation between perceived injustice and adverse recovery outcomes has been demonstrated in individuals suffering from a wide range of disabling pain conditions including whiplash injury (Scott et al., 2013), work-related low back pain (Sullivan et al., 2008), catastrophic injury (Agtarap et al., 2016), fibromyalgia (Rodero et al., 2012), sickle cell disease (Ezenwa et al., 2014), osteoarthritis (Yakobov et al., 2014), and rheumatoid arthritis (Ferrari and Russell, 2014). The pattern of findings suggests that perceptions of injustice interfere with recovery of both the physical and psychological aspects of injury. There are indications that perceptions of injustice might also play a role in the transition from acute to chronic pain following injury (Sullivan et al., 2011).

When individuals sustain a debilitating injury, their primary goals are assumed to include recovery and resumption of pre-injury involvement in various domains of their lives. It has been suggested that perceptions of injustice might lead to a reordering of the priority status of post-injury goals such that retribution goals may take precedence over recovery goals (Sullivan et al., 2014). The injured individual who adopts retribution goals has limited channels through which to inflict harm on the perceived source(s) of injustice. The injured individual consequently might resort to indirect ways of 'getting back at' perceived perpetrators. For example, retribution might take the form of expressions of criticism or irritation directed toward family members or health-care providers. Retribution aimed at health care providers might involve non-compliance with prescribed treatment or attempts to sabotage treatment altogether. Retribution aimed at an employer or insurance representative might take the form of prolonged or exaggerated disability behaviour. To the degree that the behaviours driven by retribution goals require investment of resources, these will necessarily impact negatively on the resources that can be invested in recovery or rehabilitation pursuits.

At present, little is known about the factors that give rise to perceptions of injustice. It has been suggested that perceptions of injustice are likely to emerge in situations that are characterized by a violation of basic human rights, transgressions of status or rank, or challenges to equity norms and just world beliefs (Hafer and Begue, 2005; McParland and Eccleston, 2013). Conceptual models of justice-related appraisals have highlighted the potential role of blame, loss, and suffering in the subjective experience of injustice (McParland and Eccleston 2013; Sullivan et al., 2008). Although research to date has proceeded under the assumption that perceived injustice is situation-specific, recent data suggest that individuals might also develop an enduring or characterological propensity to appraise negative events as unjust (Yakobov et al., 2019).

Health beliefs

A belief is an enduring mental representation of an idea or principle that is judged to be true. Beliefs are considered to play a significant role as determinants of decisions and behavioural choices (Fishbein and Ajzen, 1975). Health beliefs are a specific type of belief concerning individuals' mental representations of 'truth' relevant to their health (Haefner and Kirscht, 1970). In the context of musculoskeletal injury, health beliefs have been discussed as important influences on individuals' perceptions of personal vulnerability to injury, the medical and social consequences of being injured, the effectiveness of behaviours in reducing the risk of further injury, and how barriers can be overcome to adopt those behaviours (Janz and Becker, 1984).

Current empirical findings position fear-avoidance beliefs as an important type of health belief relevant to occupational engagement in individuals with musculoskeletal conditions (Schultz et al., 2002). Fear-avoidance beliefs include a conviction that prolonged rest will improve pain and disability by allowing injuries to heal, that musculoskeletal pain associated with minor physical stresses can be seriously harmful, and that neglecting pain can cause permanent health problems (Vargas-Prada and Coggon, 2015). Fear-avoidance beliefs have been assessed primarily by the Fear-Avoidance Beliefs Questionnaire (Waddell et al., 1993) and the Tampa Scale of Kinesiophobia (Kori et al., 1990). Research findings have been consistent in showing that high levels of fear-avoidance beliefs are associated with more pronounced pain-related disability (Leeuw et al., 2007).

An early study by Fritz et al. (2001) showed that high scores on a measure of fear-avoidance beliefs predicted prolonged work absence in individuals receiving physical therapy for back pain. In a sample of work-disabled individuals with musculoskeletal pain, Sullivan and Stanish (2003) reported that high levels of fear avoidance beliefs, assessed at admission, predicted lower probability of return to work after completion of a rehabilitation intervention. Sullivan et al. (2006) reported that high levels of fear avoidance beliefs contributed significant unique variance to the prediction of prolonged work absence in individuals with whiplash injuries, even when controlling for pain catastrophizing and depression. Turner et al. (2006) reported that fear avoidance beliefs were a stronger predictor of prolonged work absence than recovery expectancies in injured workers with back pain. Wideman and Sullivan (2011a) also showed that reductions in fear avoidance were associated with better return to work outcomes in injured workers with back pain. Numerous other prospective studies have shown that high scores on measures of fear avoidance beliefs impede progress and recovery through the course of rehabilitation interventions (Besen et al., 2014; Iles et al., 2008).

Psychological risk factors—mental health variables

Individuals who sustain disabling injuries are considered at risk for the development of a number of mental health problems. The bulk of research examining the relation between mental health problems and return to work outcomes has focused primarily on depression and post-traumatic stress disorder. Depression and post-traumatic stress disorder can be assessed either by diagnostic interview yielding a Diagnostic and Statistical Manual or International Classification of Diseases diagnosis, or by self-report questionnaire. In research addressing determinants of return to work, most studies have used self-report questionnaires as opposed to diagnostic interviews.

Depression

Depression is currently the leading cause of disability in industrialized countries (Friedrich, 2017). As such, disability associated with musculoskeletal injury and concurrent depression poses a particularly significant challenge, whether addressed from personal, social, occupational, or societal perspectives. Although the relation between depression and pain has been the subject of numerous investigations, only recently has research begun to specifically address the 'disability' associated with depression and pain (Sullivan et al., 2002; Turk, 2002). Symptoms of depression and pain contribute not only to suffering, but these conditions also compromise individuals' ability to participate fully in meaningful activities of their lives (Sullivan et al., 2006). Research conducted to date suggests that the presence of depressive symptoms can be considered a risk factor for prolonged work-disability following musculoskeletal injury.

Surveys indicate that approximately 20% to 50% of individuals with musculoskeletal conditions show evidence of elevated depressive symptoms (Campbell et al., 2003; Rush et al., 2000). The results of cross-sectional and prospective studies indicate that depression is associated with heightened pain and disability in patients who had sustained musculoskeletal injuries (Sullivan et al., 2002). There are also indications that the prevalence of depression might be higher in individuals who have sustained musculoskeletal injuries compared to individuals with other painful musculoskeletal conditions (Wenzel et al., 2002).

Individuals with pain-related musculoskeletal conditions and concurrent depression have sick leave duration that is twice as long as individuals with musculoskeletal conditions who are not depressed (Currie and Wang, 2004). Depressive symptoms in individuals with musculoskeletal conditions have also been associated with longer duration of wage replacement benefits following injury or surgical intervention (Cote et al., 2001; Lotters et al., 2006). Individuals with musculoskeletal conditions who present with elevated depressive symptoms are less likely to return to work following participation in a rehabilitation programme than those without depressive symptoms (Vowles et al., 2004). Depressive symptoms have been associated with premature termination of involvement in pain management programmes and greater occupational disability, and they have been implicated as contributing to the transition from acute to chronic pain (Carroll et al., 2004; Rush et al., 2000; Sullivan et al., 1992).

In many studies, depression has been shown to predict prolonged work disability even when controlling for the severity of pain symptoms (Sullivan et al., 2006). As such, depression likely impacts on pain-related disability through pathways partially distinct from those associated with pain symptoms. For example, psychomotor alterations have been associated with depression, even in the absence of pain (Sobin and Sackeim, 1997). It is possible that disability-relevant factors such as slowing of motor functions, motor initiation dysfunction, fatigue, and distress displays might be behavioural dimensions of depression that could contribute to work disability independent of pain severity.

Post-traumatic stress disorder

Post-traumatic stress disorder (PTSD) is a debilitating mental health condition that can arise following exposure to traumatic events. Common causes of PTSD include being involved in a serious motor vehicle accident, witnessing or being the victim of a violent crime, sexual abuse, military combat, and experiencing a natural disaster (Kozaric-Kovacic, 2009). PTSD is characterized by a symptom cluster that includes re-experiencing symptoms, avoidance symptoms, and symptoms of hyperarousal (APA, 2013). The risk of chronicity is significant with 11% to 44% of individuals experiencing ongoing symptoms of PTSD at 2 years after initial diagnosis (Fishbain et al., 2017; Mayou et al., 2002).

PTSD symptoms have been associated with more severe and more persistent symptoms of pain, higher levels of pain-related psychosocial risk factors, poorer physical health, and higher prevalence of comorbid mental health problems (Matthews, 2005; Sullivan et al., 2009). These sequelae or correlates of PTSD likely add to the burden of disability, in turn, compromising individuals' work potential. Symptom severity has been identified as an important predictor of work-disability in individuals with PTSD (Chossegros et al., 2011).

The symptoms of PTSD can compromise an individual's ability to participate fully in several activities of daily living. Individuals with PTSD report decreased involvement in family, social, and recreational activities (Geisser et al., 1996). Several studies have also documented a relation between PTSD and work disability. Kongsted et al. (2008) used a self-report measure of acute post-traumatic stress response following whiplash injury related to a road traffic accident to assess whether long-term occupational abilities were impacted. Indeed, moderate-to-severe levels of acute post-traumatic stress response were associated with a 2.8-fold increased risk of reduced work ability at the 1-year follow-up. Post-traumatic stress disorder 3 years following a road traffic accident was significantly associated with prolonged work absence in severely injured victims (Pelissier et al., 2017). Similarly, road accident survivors with PTSD experienced significantly more pain and had significantly less work potential at 8-months post-accident than road accident survivors without PTSD (Matthews 2005). Laisné and colleagues found that trauma symptoms were a prognostic factor in the prediction of return to work at an 8-month follow-up for individuals with work-related musculoskeletal injuries (Laisne et al., 2013).

The treatment of debilitating mental health conditions such as PTSD continues to be characterized by an overly protective orientation, where employment is viewed as an adverse stressor from which the client must be shielded, and symptom eradication is viewed as necessary before occupational resumption can be considered (Bermejo et al., 2010). Given that the symptoms of many mental health conditions can be expected to persist for extended periods of time, the pursuit of symptom eradication as a pre-condition of occupational re-engagement might contribute unnecessarily to permanent disability. Lessons learned from the treatment of musculoskeletal pain conditions suggest that successful re-engagement in occupational activities can be achieved in spite of ongoing symptoms (Sullivan and Hyman, 2014).

Implications for intervention

Evidence from a large body of prospective and longitudinal studies (see Table 9.1) points to the pivotal role of psychological variables as determinants of occupational disability in individuals with musculoskeletal injuries. Research suggests that psychological variables such as recovery expectancies, self-efficacy, pain catastrophizing, fear-avoidance beliefs, and mental health problems such as depression or PTSD contribute to prolonged work absence following musculoskeletal injury.

The results of several intervention studies further support the role of psychological variables as determinants of occupation re-engagement. Elphinston et al. (2018) showed that treatment-related changes in recovery expectancies were associated with reductions in self-rated disability. Sullivan and Stanish (2003) reported that early treatment reductions in pain catastrophizing and fear avoidance predicted successful return to work in injured workers participating in a rehabilitation intervention. The importance of reducing pain-related psychological risk factors was highlighted in a recent study where high post-treatment scores on a measure of pain catastrophizing predicted failure to maintain gains made in the rehabilitation of musculoskeletal injury (Moore et al., 2016).

Over the past two decades, great strides have been made in alerting clinicians to the importance of assessing psychological risk factors in their evaluations of individuals suffering from debilitating pain conditions. Screening measures of pain-related psychological risk factors and mental health symptomatology have been incorporated into the assessment protocols of pain clinics and rehabilitation centres around the world. Although measures of psychological risk measures have been readily adopted, the clinical community has lagged in the development and implementation of interventions specifically designed to target these psychosocial risk factors.

Cognitive-behavior theory has been the dominant conceptual framework that has guided the development of psychological interventions for individuals suffering from pain conditions. In brief, cognitive behaviour theory proposes that individuals' beliefs, interpretations, and appraisals about their pain will have a significant impact on their physical and emotional well-being (Turk, 1996). It follows that intervention techniques aimed at targeting pain-related beliefs, interpretations, and appraisals should contribute to more positive recovery outcomes.

Cognitive-behavior therapy (as applied to pain conditions) does not refer to a specific programme of treatment. Rather, cognitive-behavior therapy can best be construed as a collection of psychological or behavioural techniques with the primary objective of fostering adaptive cognitive and/or behavioural responses to pain. Cognitive-behavioral techniques vary widely in their characteristics and their intended impact. Some techniques are aimed at reducing the severity of physical or emotional symptoms, others at promoting re-engagement in important life activities, and still others at fostering more effective self-management. Some techniques might be combined into a structured programme of treatment, while others might be delivered as brief stand-alone interventions.

The variability in content and focus of cognitive-behavioural interventions for pain presents challenges with respect to describing cognitive-behavioural interventions, and for making statements about the their effectiveness. Another complicating factor

Table 9.1 Table of studies

Citation	Study design	Occupational engagement outcome	Sample	Duration of follow-up	Outcome
Adams, H. et al., Psychosocial factors related to return to work following rehabilitation of whiplash injuries. *J Occup Rehabil.* 2007; 17(2), 305–315.	Prospective Cohort Study	RTW	75 work-disabled individuals with a diagnosis of Whiplash Grade II	10 weeks	Treatment-related reductions in catastrophizing, fear of movement and pain intensity were associated with RTW. Self-reported disability was found particularly resistant to change as the period of work disability extends over time.
Adams H. et al., The relation between catastrophizing and occupational disability in individuals with major depression: Concurrent and prospective associations. *J Occup Rehabil.* 2017;27:405–12.	Prospective Cohort Study	RTW, measured using days of absence, days of limitation, and work status	80 work-disabled individuals with major depressive disorder (MDD)	1 month	Reductions in catastrophic thinking predicted successful RTW following rehabilitation intervention, beyond the variance accounted for by reductions in depressive symptom severity.
Besan E. et al., Returning to work following low back pain: Towards a model of individual psychosocial factors. *J Occup Rehabil.* 2015; 25(1): 25–37.	Prospective Cohort Study and Model Development	RTW, measured using days of absence, days of limitation, and work status	241 individuals with work-related low back pain (injury <14 days old)	3 months	Fear avoidance beliefs had a significant indirect influence on RTW: Fear avoidance beliefs impacted RTW expectations, which in turn impacted on days of absence, days of limitation, and work status.

Boersma K. and Linton S. J. Screening to identify patients at risk—Profiles of psychological risk factors for early intervention. *Clin J Pain*, 2005; 21:38–43	Prospective Cohort Study	Long-term sick leave (>15 days)	363 individuals with acute/subacute nonspecific neck or back pain	1 year	Individuals with high scores on all variables (pain intensity, depressed mood, fear-avoidance, and function) were much more likely to have been on long-term sick leave at the 1-year follow-up. Individuals with high scores on all variables except depressed mood were also likely to have been on long-term sick leave at the 1-year follow-up, but much less so.
Bostick G. P. et al., Predictive capacity of pain beliefs and catastrophizing in whiplash associated disorder. *Injury* 2013;44:1456–71.	Prospective Cohort Study	Self-reported disability	72 individuals undergoing treatment for acute whiplash injury	3 and 6 months	Health beliefs related to permanence and mysteriousness of pain and catastrophizing were predictive of future disability.
Brede E. et al., Prediction of failure to retain work 1 year after interdisciplinary functional restoration in occupational injuries. *Arch Phys Med Rehabil.* 2012; 93:268–74.	Prospective Cohort Study	Employment stability (ability to retain work)	1850 individuals with musculoskeletal injuries, disabled for >4 months	1 year	Individuals with pre-treatment BDI scores above a clinical cut score (equal to or above 20) were less likely to have returned to work at the 1-year follow-up.
Brouwer S. et al., A prospective study of return to work across health conditions: Perceived work attitude, self-efficacy and perceived social support. *J Occup Rehabil.* 2010; 20:104–12.	Prospective Cohort Study	RTW	352 individuals with back- or limb-related musculoskeletal conditions on sickness absence	10 months	Perceived work attitude, perceived social support, and self-efficacy were relevant predictors with regard to the time to RTW.

(continued)

Table 9.1 Table of studies (*continued*)

Citation	Study design	Occupational engagement outcome	Sample	Duration of follow-up	Outcome
Burton A. K. et al., Psychosocial predictors of outcome in acute and subchronic low back trouble. *Spine (Phila Pa 1976)*. 1995 15; 20(6):722–8.	Prospective Cohort Study	Self-reported disability, including occupational disability	250 individuals with LBP	1 year	Pain locus of control, coping strategies, depression, somatic perception, and fear-avoidance beliefs were associated with future disability. Catastrophizing was found almost 7 times more important than clinical and historical variables for the acute cases.
Busch, H. et al., Self-efficacy beliefs predict sustained long-term sick absenteeism in individuals with chronic musculoskeletal pain. *Pain Pract*. 2007; 7(3), 234–40.	Prospective Cohort Study	Sustained long-term sick absenteeism	223 individuals with nonspecific chronic musculoskeletal disorders	1 year	Subjects with negative recovery beliefs, low sense of mastery, perceived high mental demands at work, and prior experiences of long-term sick absenteeism had an increased probability of receiving sickness benefits at follow-up. Prolonged sickness absence contributed strongly to increase individuals' sense of helplessness, lower self-efficacy, and hindered future work return.
Carriere J. S. et al., Expectancies mediate the relationship between perceived injustice and return to work following whiplash injury: A 1-year prospective study. *Eur J Pain*. 2017; 21:1234–42.	Prospective Cohort Study	Work status; RTW expectancies	152 individuals with a primary diagnosis of whiplash injury	1 year	High scores on measure of perceived injustice were associated with prolonged work disability. High perceptions of injustice were associated with low return-to-work expectancies.

Reference	Study design	Outcome	Sample	Follow-up	Findings
Carriere J. S. et al., The mediating role of recovery expectancies on the relation between depression and return-to-work. *J Occup Rehabil.* 2015; 25:348–56	Prospective Cohort Study	RTW	109 individuals with work-related musculoskeletal disorders and depressive symptoms	1 year	Lower recovery expectancies and depressive symptoms were associated with a lower probability of RTW. Recovery expectancies were found to mediate the relation between depression and RTW status at 1-year follow-up.
Chossegros L. et al., Predictive factors of chronic post-traumatic stress disorder 6 months after a road traffic accident. *Accid Anal Prev.* 2011; 43:471–7.	Prospective Cohort Study	RTW	592 individuals injured in a road traffic accident	6 months	Participants with more PTSD symptoms had more difficulty returning to work after the accident.
Cole D. C. et al., Listening to injured workers: How recovery expectations predict outcomes--a prospective study. *CMAJ.* 2002 19; 166:749–54.	Prospective Cohort Study	Cumulative days receiving 100% wage replacement benefits	1566 individuals with soft-tissue injury to back or extremities	1 year	Injured individuals' expectations of slower recovery were consistently associated with longer duration of time loss claims.
Cote P.S. et al., The association between neck pain intensity, physical functioning, depressive symptomatology and time-to-claim-closure after whiplash. *J Clin Epidemiol.* 2001; 54:275–86.	Prospective Cohort Study	Time-to-claim-closure	5398 individuals having submitted claims due to whiplash injury	1 year	The presence of depressive symptomatology reduced the claim-closure rate by 36%. Lower pain, better function, and the absence of depressive symptoms were found strongly associated with faster time-to-claim-closure and recovery after whiplash, independent of the insurance system.

(continued)

Table 9.1 Table of studies (*continued*)

Citation	Study design	Occupational engagement outcome	Sample	Duration of follow-up	Outcome
Currie S.R. and Wang J.L. Chronic back pain and major depression in the general Canadian population. *Pain*. 2004; 107:54–60.	Cross-sectional Study	Number of disability days in past 2 weeks	Subsample of individuals (n = 10 600; 9% of sample) with chronic back pain from population survey	n/a	High scores of depressive symptoms was associated with increased reporting of some disability days in the past 2 weeks.
Dionne, C.E., et al., Determinants of 'return to work in good health' among workers with back pain who consult in primary care settings: A 2-year prospective study. *Eur Spine J*. 2007; 16, 641–55.	Prospective Cohort Study	Return to work in good health (RWGH)	1007 individuals with non-specific back pain	24 months	High self-efficacy was associated with success in RWGH. Fear-avoidance beliefs were associated with failure.
Dozois D.J.A. et al., Factors associated with rehabilitation outcome in patients with low back pain (LBP): Prediction of employment outcome at 9-month follow-up. *Rehabil Psychol*. 1995; 40: 243–59.	Prospective Cohort Study	RTW	117 males with LBP	10 months	Higher scores on a measure of depressive symptoms was associated with lower rates of RTW at follow-up.

Druss B. G. et al., Health and disability costs of depressive illness in a major U.S. corporation. *Am J Psychiatry*. 2000; 157:1274–8.	Cross-sectional Study	Health care cost; sick days	15 153 individuals working at a major US corporation who filed health claims	n/a	Individuals experiencing both depression and a medical problem, such as back pain, had health costs that were over 2 times higher and 1.5–2× more sick days than individuals only experiencing depression or a medical problem.
Du Bois M. and Donceel P. A screening questionnaire to predict no return to work within 3 months for low back pain claimants. *Eur Spine J*. 2008; 17:380–5.	Prospective Cohort Study	RTW	186 individuals with LBP submitting a claim for sickness benefits to social health insurance	3 months	Work-disabled individuals who were less than 100% certain that they would RTW within the next 6 months, were 4 times less likely to RTW during that time period.
Du Bois M., Szpalski M., and Donceel P. Patients at risk for long-term sick leave because of low back pain. *Spine J*. 2009; 9: 350–9.	Prospective Cohort Study	RTW	346 disabled individuals with LBP applying for compensation benefits	3 months	Fear of avoidance scores were considered a risk factor for RTW at 3 months.
Fritz J. M. and George S. Z. Identifying psychosocial variables in patients with acute work-related low back pain: The importance of fear-avoidance beliefs. *Phys Ther*. 2002; 82:973–83.	Prospective Cohort Study	RTW	78 people with acute/subacute work-related low back pain	4 weeks	The work subscale of the Fear-Avoidance Beliefs Questionnaire was the strongest predictor of RTW.
Fritz J. M. et al., The role of fear-avoidance beliefs in acute low back pain: Relationships with current and future disability and work status. *Pain*. 2001; 94:7–15.	Prospective Cohort Study	RTW	78 people with acute/subacute work-related low back pain	4 weeks	The work subscale of the Fear-Avoidance Beliefs Questionnaire significantly contributed to the prediction of RTW.

(continued)

Table 9.1 Table of studies (*continued*)

Citation	Study design	Occupational engagement outcome	Sample	Duration of follow-up	Outcome
Gallagher R. M. et al., Determinants of return-to-work among low back pain patients. *Pain.* 1989; 39:55–67.	Prospective Cohort Study	RTW	150 individuals with LBP	6 months	Medical and physical features alone failed to adequately predict disability. Accurate predictions considered a myriad of psychosocial variables and adjusted for age and time out of work.
Gauthier N. et al., Investigating risk factors for chronicity: The importance of distinguishing between return-to-work status and self-report measures of disability. *J Occup Environ Med.* 2006; 48:312–8.	Prospective Cohort Study	RTW	255 claimants of a worker's compensation board, off work for min. 6 weeks due to a soft tissue back injury sustained in an occupational incident with at least 1 'yellow flag' (described in text)	4 weeks after termination of treatment program	Higher scores on a measure of pain catastrophizing was predictive of reduced likelihood in having RTW at follow-up.
Gheldolf E. L. M. et al., The differential role of pain, work characteristics and pain-related fear in explaining back pain and sick leave in occupational settings. *Pain.* 2005; 113:71–81.	Cross-sectional Study	Short- (1–30 days in past year) and long-term (>30 days in past year) sick leave	1294 working individuals with and without LBP	n/a	Both short- and long-term sick leave were strongly associated with fear of movement and (re)injury.

Reference	Study type	Outcome	Sample	Follow-up	Findings
Giummarra, M.J. et al., Return to work after traumatic injury: Increased work-related disability in injured persons receiving financial compensation is mediated by perceived injustice. *J Occup Rehabil.* 2017; 27: 173.	Prospective Cohort Study	Receiving compensation; RTW	364 individuals with diverse traumatic injuries recruited from the Victorian State Trauma Registry	1 year	Perceived injustice and distress symptoms led to a twofold to sevenfold increase in the risk of failing to RTW. Anxiety, post-traumatic stress, and perceived injustice were elevated following compensable injury compared with non-compensable injury.
Hagen E.M. et al., Predictors and modifiers of treatment effect influencing sick leave in subacute low back pain patients. *Spine.* 2006; 30. 2717–23.	Prospective Cohort Study	RTW	457 individuals sick-listed 8 to 12 weeks for LBP	1 year	The belief that work would aggravate the condition was a significant predictor of non-RTW at 3 months, whereas the lack of belief that back pain would disappear was a significant predictor of non-RTW at 1 year. Belief that work would aggravate the condition and self-reported disability complaints were associated with longer sick leave.
Haldorsen E. M. H. et al., Patients with low back pain not returning to work: A 12-month follow-up study. *Spine.* 1998; 23:1202–8.	Prospective Cohort Study	RTW	260 individuals with LBP	1 year	For those not returning to work, low internal health locus of control score, restricted lateral mobility, and reduced work ability were predictive variables in combination.
Hallegraeff J. M. et al., Expectations about recovery from acute non-specific low back pain predict absence from usual work due to chronic low back pain: A systematic review. *J Physiother.* 2012; 58:165–72.	Prospective Cohort Study	RTW	241 individuals with LBP	3 months	Individuals with low recovery expectancies were more than twice as likely to be work-disabled than those with high recovery expectancies.

(continued)

Table 9.1 Table of studies (*continued*)

Citation	Study design	Occupational engagement outcome	Sample	Duration of follow-up	Outcome
Klenerman L. et al., The prediction of chronicity in patients with an acute attack of low back pain in a general practice setting. *Spine*. 1995; 20:478–84.	Prospective Cohort Study	Sick leave	300 individuals experiencing an episode of acute LBP	1 year	Fear-avoidance significantly predicted sick leave and correctly classified 70% of individuals with regards to sick leave.
Kongsted A. T. et al., Acute stress response and recovery after whiplash injuries. A one-year prospective study. *Eur J Pain*. 2008; 12:455–63.	Prospective Cohort Study	Ability to work ('unaffected', 'reduced working ability', or 'off sick')	668 individuals with acute whiplash	1 year	Acute stress response (as measured by the IES-R) was associated with RTW.
Lackner J. M. et al., Pain expectancies, pain, and functional self-efficacy expectancies as determinants of disability in patients with chronic low back disorders. *J Consult Clin Psychol*. 1996; 64:212–20.	Cross-sectional Study	Abilities to perform essential job tasks (functional self-efficacy (FSE))	85 individuals with a variety of chronic low back disorders and injuries	n/a	FSE was significantly related to functional performance when re-injury and pain were partialed out. Performance-specific cognitions related to work had greater explanatory power over disability than pain-specific ones.
Laisne F. et al., Biopsychosocial determinants of work outcomes of workers with occupational injuries receiving compensation: A prospective study. *Work*. 2013; 44:117–32.	Prospective Cohort Study	Involved in RTW process	62 individuals with work-related musculoskeletal injuries	2 and 8 months	Individuals with more PTSD symptoms were less likely to be engaged in the RTW process at the 8-month follow-up, but not the 2-month follow-up.

Lotters F. et al., The prognostic value of depressive symptoms, fear-avoidance, and self-efficacy for duration of lost-time benefits in workers with musculoskeletal disorders. *Occup Environ Med.* 2006; 63:794–801.	Prospective Cohort Study	Total compensation benefit	187 individuals receiving total compensation benefits due to musculoskeletal disorders	1 year	Increased depressive symptoms significantly increased the number of days on total benefit.
Lotters F. and Burdorf A. Prognostic factors for duration of sickness absence due to musculoskeletal disorders. *Clin J Pain.* 2006; 22:212–21.	Prospective Cohort Study	Sickness absence	253 individuals with musculoskeletal disorders and on sick leave for 2 to 6 weeks	1 year	For individuals with LBP, perception of one's inability to RTW was predictive of longer sickness absence.
Matthews L. R. Work potential of road accident survivors with post-traumatic stress disorder. *Behav Res Ther.* 2005; 43:475–83.	Cross-sectional Study	Work Potential Profile (self-report questionnaire)	46 road accident survivors	n/a	Individuals with PTSD scored lower on the Work Potential Profile than individuals without PTSD.
Pélisier C. et al., Factors associated with non-return to work in the severely injured victim 3 years after a road accident—A prospective study. *Accid Anal Prev.* 2017; 106:411–9.	Cross-sectional Study	RTW	224 severely injured road accident victims (M-AIS > or = 3)	3 years	PTSD was associated with non-return to work at the 3-year follow-up, and acted as an essential modifiable medical determinant in returning to work.
Richard S. et al., Self-efficacy and health locus of control: Relationship to occupational disability among workers with back pain. *J Occup Rehabil.* 2011; 21:421–30.	Prospective Cohort Study	Return to work in good health (RWGH)	1,007 individuals with occupational disruptions due to nonspecific back pain	24 months	Higher scores on the self-efficacy questionnaire were protective of 'failure to return to work after attempt(s)' and of 'failure to return to work'.

(continued)

Table 9.1 Table of studies (continued)

Citation	Study design	Occupational engagement outcome	Sample	Duration of follow-up	Outcome
Sarda J. et al., The contribution of self-efficacy and depression to disability and work status in chronic pain patients: A comparison between Australian and Brazilian samples. *Eur J Pain.* 2009; 13:189–95.	Cross-sectional Study	Working status	622 individuals experiencing chronic pain (311 from Australia and 311 from Brazil)	n/a	Different factors were relevant in predicting work status in the two populations: self-efficacy contributed to the prediction of work status in the Brazilian sample, whereas depression contributed to the prediction of work status in the Australian population.
Schade V. et al., The impact of clinical, morphological, psychosocial and work-related factors on the outcome of lumbar discectomy. *Pain.* 1999; 80:239–49.	Prospective Cohort Study	RTW	42 consecutive individuals with a symptomatic disc herniation undergoing a lumbar discectomy	23–30 months	High levels of depression had a negative influence on RTW, and depression was a significant predictor of RTW.
Schultz I. Z. et al., Predicting return to work after low back injury using the psychosocial risk for occupational disability instrument: A validation study. *J Occup Rehabil.* 2005; 15:365–76.	Cross-sectional Study	RTW	100 individuals with LBP who have been work-disabled for 4–6 weeks	3 months	Expectations of recovery, quality of life, and mental health variables predicted RTW outcomes in the subacute stage after LBP injury. There were significant differences in scores on psychological health between RTW group and non-RTW group.

Reference	Study type	Outcomes	Sample	Follow-up	Findings
Schultz I. Z. et al., Psychosocial factors predictive of occupational low back disability—Towards development of a return-to-work model. *Pain*. 2004; 107:77–85.	Prospective Cohort Study	Return to Work status; Duration of disability; Disability costs	253 subacute and chronic pain injured individuals with non-specific low back injuries	RTW status: 3 months after first evaluation All other outcomes: 18 months after injury	The key psychosocial predictors identified were expectations of recovery and perception of health change. Also implicated, but to a lesser degree, were occupational stability, skill discretion at work, co-worker support, and the response of the individuals' compensation system and employer to the disability.
Scott W. Z. et al., Further validation of a measure of injury-related injustice perceptions to identify risk for occupational disability: A prospective study of individuals with whiplash injury. *J Occup Rehabil*. 2013; 23:557–65.	Prospective Cohort Study	RTW	103 whiplash-injured individuals	1 year	Scores on perceived injustice significantly discriminated individuals who returned and did not RTW at the follow-up. Examination of specific scores revealed that a post-treatment score of greater than 19 optimally identified individuals who had returned to work from those who had not.
Scott W. Z. et al., Barriers to change in depressive symptoms following multidisciplinary rehabilitation for whiplash: The role of perceived injustice. *Clin J Pain*. 2015; 31:145–51.	Prospective Cohort Study	Sick leave	53 individuals with whiplash injury and depressive symptoms	7 weeks	Longer work absence and greater perceived injustice predicted worse improvement in depressive symptoms. Greater perceived injustice was also associated with persistence of clinically significant depressive symptoms at post-treatment stage.

(continued)

Table 9.1 Table of studies (*continued*)

Citation	Study design	Occupational engagement outcome	Sample	Duration of follow-up	Outcome
Soderlund A. and Asenlof P. The mediating role of self-efficacy expectations and fear of movement and (re)injury beliefs in two samples of acute pain. *Disabil Rehabil.* 2010; 32:2118–26.	Cross-sectional Study	Pain-related disability	64 individuals with acute whiplash-associated disorders (WAD) and 74 individuals with nonspecific musculoskeletal injury	n/a	In individuals with WAD, low self-efficacy and intense pain predicted disability. In individuals with MSI, kinesophobia and intense pain predicted disability.
Sullivan M.J.L. and Stanish W.D. Psychologically based occupational rehabilitation: The pain-disability prevention program. *Clin J Pain.* 2003; 19:97–104.	Prospective Cohort Study	RTW	104 claimants of a worker's compensation board, off work for min. 6 weeks due to a back injury with at least 1 'yellow flag' (described in text)	Upon treatment completion (maximum of 10 weeks after beginning treatment)	Pre-treatment scores on the BDI-II predicted RTW.

Reference	Study Design	Outcome	Sample	Duration	Findings
Sullivan M. J. et al., Catastrophizing, pain, and disability in patients with soft-tissue injuries. *Pain.* 1998; 77:253–60.	Cross-sectional Study	Employment Status	86 individuals with soft-tissue injuries to the neck, shoulders or back following work or motor vehicle accidents.	n/a	Depression (as measured by the BDI) was significantly associated with the occupation item of the Pain Disability Index. Catastrophizing was significantly correlated with individuals' reported pain intensity, perceived disability and employment status. Catastrophizing contributed to the prediction of disability over and above the variance accounted for by pain intensity and independent of the levels of depression and anxiety.
Sullivan M. J. et al., Differential predictors of pain and disability in patients with whiplash injuries. *Pain Res Manag.* 2002; 7:68–74.	Cross-sectional Study	Perceived Disability	65 individuals with whiplash injuries	n/a	Psychological variables together accounted for 18% of the variance in pain rating and 37% of the variance in perceived disability scores.
Sullivan M. J. et al., Secondary prevention of work disability: Community-based psychosocial intervention for musculoskeletal disorders. *J Occup Rehabil.* 2005; 15:377–92.	Prospective Cohort Study	RTW	215 work-disabled individuals with musculoskeletal injury	4 weeks	Treatment reductions in catastrophic thinking improved probability of RTW.
Sullivan M.J.L. et al., A psychosocial risk factor-targeted intervention for the prevention of chronic pain and disability following whiplash injury. *Phys Ther.* 2006; 86:8–18.	Prospective Cohort Study	RTW	70 individuals with sustained whiplash injuries	10 weeks	Inclusion of the Progressive Goal Attainment Program (PGAP) intervention significantly increased the likelihood of RTW, and individuals who presented with more psychosocial risk factors were more likely to benefit from PGAP.

(continued)

Table 9.1 Table of studies (*continued*)

Citation	Study design	Occupational engagement outcome	Sample	Duration of follow-up	Outcome
Sullivan M.J.L. et al., Stage of chronicity and treatment response in patients with musculoskeletal injuries and concurrent symptoms of depression. *Pain.* 2008;135:151–9.	Prospective Cohort Study	RTW	80 individuals with disabling musculoskeletal conditions and concurrent depressive symptoms	4 weeks after termination of treatment program	Change in depression scores (as measured by the BDI-II) partially mediated the relationship between chronicity and RTW.
Sullivan, M.J.L. et al., The role of perceived injustice in the experience of chronic pain and disability: Scale development and validation. *J Occup Rehabil.* 2008; 18(3), 249–261.	Prospective Cohort Study	RTW	226 individuals with musculoskeletal conditions	1 year	High scores on a measure of perceived injustice were related to less rehabilitation progress and lower probability of RTW following musculoskeletal injury.
Sullivan M.J. et al., Pain, perceived injustice and the persistence of post-traumatic stress symptoms during the course of rehabilitation for whiplash injuries. *Pain.* 2009; 145:325–31.	Cross-sectional Study	Functional disability	85 individuals with whiplash injuries	n/a	High levels of perceived injustice were associated with more intense pain, higher levels of catastrophic thinking, depression, and disability. Individuals with high levels of perceived injustice displayed more protective pain behaviours than individuals with low levels of perceived injustice, regardless of the level of physical demand of the task.

Citation	Study Design	Outcome	Sample	Follow-up	Findings
Sullivan M.J.L. et al., Report R-675. Pain, depression, disability, and rehabilitation outcomes. 2006. https://www.irsst.qc.ca/media/documents/PubIRSST/R-675.pdf	Prospective Cohort Study	RTW	207 individuals with musculoskeletal injuries	1 year	Depressed individuals were less likely to RTW than non-depressed individuals, and of the individuals that did RTW, depressed individuals were less likely to be working full-time. Pre-treatment depression scores significantly predicted RTW.
Thompson D. P. et al., Cognitive determinants of pain and disability in patients with chronic whiplash-associated disorder—A cross-sectional observational study. Physiotherapy. 2010; 96:151–159.	Cross-sectional Study	Disability	55 individuals with chronic Whiplash-Associated Disorder	n/a	Greater catastrophising and lower functional self-efficacy beliefs predicted greater levels of disability.
Truchon M. et al., Low-back-pain related disability: An integration of psychological risk factors into the stress process model. Pain. 2008; 137:564–73.	Cross-sectional Study	Functional Disability	439 individuals with LBP-related disability	n/a	A model relating life events, cognitive appraisal, emotional distress, and avoidance coping to functional disability was validated.
Turner J. A. et al., Worker recovery expectations and fear-avoidance predict work disability in a population-based workers' compensation back pain sample. Spine (Phila Pa 1976). 2006 ; 31:682–9.	Prospective Cohort Study	Work disability	1068 individuals with work-related back pain	6 months	Injured individuals who reported 'low certainty' of RTW within the next 6 months had over 12 times the number of disability days than those who were 'extremely certain' of returning to work. High, moderate, and low scores about work fear avoidance beliefs (using the work fear avoidance subscale of the Fear-Avoidance Beliefs Questionnaire) were significantly predictive of work disability.

(continued)

Table 9.1 Table of studies (*continued*)

Citation	Study design	Occupational engagement outcome	Sample	Duration of follow-up	Outcome
Van der Giezen A. et al., Prediction of return-to-work of low back pain patients sicklisted for 3–4 months. *Pain.* 2000; 87:285–94.	Prospective Cohort Study	RTW	328 individuals on sick leave due to LBP	1 year	Health beliefs were related to less rehabilitation progress and lower probability of RTW.
Verbunt J. A. et al., A new episode of low back pain: Who relies on bed rest? *Eur J Pain.* 2008; 12:508–16.	Prospective Cohort Study	Work disability	282 individuals with non-specific LBP	1 year	Catastrophizing and fear of injury predicted prolonged bed rest more than pain history or pain intensity. Longer bed rest in the early stages of injury may precipitate long term disability.
Vowles K. E. et al., Predicting work status following interdisciplinary treatment for chronic pain. *Eur J Pain.* 2004; 8:351–8.	Cross-sectional Study	RTW	138 individuals with chronic pain	n/a	Depression, as measured by BDI-II, was one of the best predictors of post-treatment work status.
Wideman T. H. and Sullivan M.J.L. Differential predictors of the long-term levels of pain intensity, work disability, healthcare use, and medication use in a sample of worker's compensation claimants. *Pain.* 2011; 152:376–83.	Prospective Cohort Study	RTW	235 individuals with subacute work-related back or neck injury receiving wage indemnity benefits	1 year	Fear avoidance beliefs predicted RTW status at 1-year follow-up.
Wideman T. H. and Sullivan M.J.L. Development of a cumulative psychosocial factor index for problematic recovery following work-related musculoskeletal injuries. *Phys Ther.* 2012; 91:1–1.1	Prospective Cohort Study	RTW	235 individuals with subacute work-related back or neck injury receiving wage indemnity benefits	1 year	The more psychological risk factors (depression, catastrophizing, fear) were presented, the less likely an individual was to RTW.

Note: BDI, Beck Depression Inventory; LBP, low-back pain; RTW, Return to work.

is that cognitive-behavioural interventions are often included as one component of multipronged or multidisciplinary treatment programmes for chronic pain. While cognitively oriented multidisciplinary pain programmes have been shown to be effective, it is difficult to evaluate the specific contribution of the psychological components of these programmes.

A recent review of research examining the effectiveness of cognitive-behaviour interventions on the reduction of pain catastrophizing revealed only modest effects (Schutze et al., 2018). The authors of the review questioned whether observed effects were of sufficient magnitude to be of clinical relevance. Similarly, two studies of the outcomes of multidisciplinary pain programmes revealed negligible effects on perceptions of injustice (Scott et al., 2013; Sullivan et al., 2008). It is possible that current 'untargeted' application of cognitive behavioural approaches to the management of pain-related disability might not yield reductions in psychological risk factors of sufficient magnitude to positively influence return to work outcomes. A more targeted approach might need to be considered. In other words, if specific psychological variables have been linked to problematic recovery outcomes, the most effective interventions might be those that contain techniques specifically designed to reduce these psychological variables.

Research on psychological risk factors for prolonged pain and disability has prompted the development of risk-factor targeted intervention for pain-related disability. For example, risk-targeted behavioural activation interventions have been shown to yield substantive reductions in pain catastrophizing in individuals suffering from a range of pain conditions such as back pain, whiplash, and fibromyalgia (Sullivan and Adams 2010; Sullivan et al., 2012; Sullivan et al., 2006). In turn, treatment-related reductions in pain catastrophizing have been associated with improved return-to-work outcomes. Techniques used to target catastrophizing include guided disclosure, validation, goal setting, emotional problem solving, and activity scheduling (Wideman and Sullivan, 2011b).

Targeted exposure interventions have also shown promise in reducing psychological risk factors for pain-related disability. According to the Fear-Avoidance Model, individuals differ in the degree to which they interpret their pain symptoms in a 'catastrophic' or 'alarmist' manner. The model predicts that catastrophic thinking following the onset of pain will contribute to heightened fears of movement. In turn, fear is expected to lead to avoidance of activity that might be associated with pain (Vlaeyen and Linton, 2000). According to the Fear-Avoidance Model, reducing fear of movement is a critical component of successful rehabilitation of individuals with debilitating pain conditions. Exposure to feared activities is a treatment approach that involves systematic exposure or engagement in activities that individuals avoid due to fears that they might experience an exacerbation of their symptoms. Exposure interventions aimed at reducing fear of movement have been shown to be effective in reducing disability, reducing absenteeism, and facilitating return to work (Bailey et al., 2010; Vlaeyen et al., 2001).

There has been little advance on interventions designed to modify recovery expectancies, self-efficacy, or perceptions of injustice. There are currently no intervention programmes that have been developed specifically to modify recovery expectancies, self-efficacy, or perceptions of injustice. Furthermore, the current state of knowledge provides little guidance about the nature of interventions that would be required to effectively modify these psychological risk factors. Little is currently known about the determinants of recovery expectancies, self-efficacy, or perceived injustice following musculoskeletal injury. As well, little is known about the determinants of changes in recovery expectancies, self-efficacy, or perceived injustice. These knowledge gaps will necessarily impede efforts to develop evidence-informed approaches to modifying psychological risk factors for prolonged work disability.

Although numerous treatment approaches have been developed to reduce the severity of symptoms of depression and PTSD, the degree to which these treatments influence return to work outcomes remains unclear. Certain antidepressants used in the treatment of depression and PTSD have sedating effects that risk increasing rather than decreasing disability, particularly if combined with opiate analgesics. The current interest in using medicinal cannabinoids for the treatment of PTSD might also inadvertently contribute to an increase in disability. The disabling nature of symptom-focused interventions is a topic that deserves more research and clinical reflection.

Summary

Research over the past two decades a pointed to a number of pain-related psychological variables and mental health conditions that impede recovery following musculoskeletal injury. This chapter briefly reviewed evidence suggesting that pain-related psychological variables such as recovery expectancies, self-efficacy, pain catastrophizing, perceived injustice, and fear-avoidance beliefs play a significant role as determinants of work-disability in individuals with musculoskeletal conditions. Research was also reviewed showing that mental health problems such as depression and PTSD also contribute to prolonged work disability in individuals with musculoskeletal conditions. The strength of the findings makes a strong case for recommending assessment of pain-related psychological variables, depression, and PTSD when planning treatment for individuals with musculoskeletal conditions.

There are important knowledge gaps that will need to be addressed in order to improve treatment outcomes for individuals presenting with a psychological risk profile. First, it is not clear that variables such as recovery expectancies, self-efficacy, pain catastrophizing, perceived injustice, and fear-avoidance beliefs contribute 'unique' variance to the prediction of problematic recovery outcomes. Available research suggests significant variance overlap among these measures. Few prospective studies have been conducted where more than one or two of these variables are assessed concurrently. A pain-related psychological variable could emerge as predictor of problematic outcomes when tested in isolation, but not when competing with other possible risk factors. The realities of clinical practice place limits on the number of questionnaires that can be included in assessment protocols. Identification of the key psychological variables impacting on recovery outcomes would permit streamlining assessment protocols of focus on variables with the highest predictive values. In addition, research examining the relative importance of different pain-related psychological risk factors might also help identify key targets for psychosocial interventions designed to improve recovery trajectories following musculoskeletal injury.

Available evidence suggests that current cognitive behavioural approaches to modifying pain-related psychological risk factors might be yielding effects of insufficient magnitude to impact in a meaningful manner on clinical outcomes. Although numerous studies have shown statistically significant changes in pain-related psychological risk factors, the clinical significance of observed changes has been questioned. With respect to depression and PTSD, more research is needed to improve the functional outcomes of treatment. While many treatments have been shown to be effective in yielding reductions in depression and PTSD, it is not clear that symptom reduction has been sufficient to improve return work outcomes. In many domains of research, symptom reduction has not been shown to be a necessary or sufficient condition for successful return to work. Excessive focus on symptom reduction might inadvertently contribute to increases rather than decreases in work-disability.

References

Aceves-Avila, F. J., Ferrari, R., and Ramos-Remus, C. (2004). New insights into culture driven disorders. *Best Practice & Research. Clinical Rheumatology,* **18,** 55–171.

Agtarap, S., Scott, W., Warren, A. M., and Trost, Z. (2016) Validation of the Injustice Experiences Questionnaire in a heterogeneous trauma sample. *Rehabilitation Psychology,* **61,** 336–44.

APA. (2013) *Diagnostic and Statistical Manual of Mental Disorders.* 5th edn. Arlington, VA: American Psychiatric Publishing.

Bailey, K., Carleton, N., Vlaeyen, J. W. S., and Asmundson, G. J. (2010) Treatments addressing pain-related fear and anxiety in patients with chronic musculoskeletal pain: A preliminary review. *Cognitive Behavior Therapy,* **39,** 46–63.

Bandura, A. (1977) *Self-Efficacy: The Exercise of Control.* New York: Freeman.

Barry, L. C., Guo, Z., Kerns, R. D., Duong, B. D., and Reid, M. C. (2003) Functional self-efficacy and pain-related disability among older veterans with chronic pain in a primary care setting. *Pain,* **104,** 131–37.

Bergbom, S., Boersma, K., Overmeer, T., and Linton, S. J. (2011) Relationship among pain catastrophizing, depressed mood, and outcomes across physical therapy treatments. *Physical Therapy,* **91,** 754–64.

Bermejo, I., Kriston, L., Schneider, F., Gaebel, W., Hegerl, U., Berger, M., and Harter, M. (2010) Sick leave and depression—determining factors and clinical effect in outpatient care. *Psychiatry Research,* **180,** 68–73.

Besen, E., Young, A. E., and Shaw, W. S. (2015) Returning to work following low back pain: Towards a model of individual psychosocial factors. *Journal of Occupational Rehabilitation,* 25, 25–37.

Brouwer, S., Amick, B. C., Lee, H., Franche, R. L., Hogg-Johnson, S. (2015) The predictive validity of the Return-to-Work Self-Efficacy Scale for return-to-work outcomes in claimants with musculoskeletal disorders. *Journal of Occupational Rehabilitation,* 25, 725–32.

Brouwer, S., Reneman, M. F., Bultman, U., ven der Klink, J. J. L. and Groothoff, J. W. (2011) A prospective study of return to work across health conditions: Perceived work attitude, self-efficacy and perceived social support., *Journal of Occupational Rehabilitation,* 20, 104–12.

Burton, A. K., Tittotson, K. M., Main, C. J., and Hollis, S. (1995) Psychological predictors of outcome in acute and subchronic low back trouble. *Spine*, **20**, 722–8.

Campbell, L. C., Clauw, D. J., and Keefe, F. J. (2003) Persistent pain and depression: A biopsychoscial perspective. *Biological Psychiatry*, **54**, 399–409.

Carriere, J. S., Thibault, P., Adams, H., Milioto, M., Ditto, B., and Sullivan, M. J. L. (2017) Expectancies mediate the relationship between perceived injustice and return to work following whiplash injury: A 1-year prospective study, *European Journal of Pain*, **21**, 1234–42.

Carriere, J. S., Thibault, P., and Sullivan, M. J. (2015a) The mediating role of recovery expectancies on the relation between depression and return-to-work. *Journal of Occupational Rehabilitation*, **25**, 348–56.

Carriere, J. S., Thibault, P., Milioto, M., and Sullivan, M. J. L. (2015b) Expectancies mediate the relations among pain catastrophizing, fear of movement, and return to work after whiplash injury. *Journal of Pain*, **16**, 1280–7.

Carroll, L. J., Cassidy, J. D., and Cote, P. (2004) Depression as a risk factor for onset of an episode of troublesome neck and low back pain. *Pain*, **107**, 134–9.

Carroll, L. J., Lis, A., Weiser, S., and Torti, J. (2016) How well do you expect to recover, and what does recovery mean, anyway? Qualitative study of expectations after a musculoskeletal injury. *Physical Therapy*, **96**, 797–807.

Chossegros, L., Hours, M., Charnay, P., Bernard, M., Fort, E., Boisson, D., et al. (2011) Predictive factors of chronic post-traumatic stress disorder 6 months after a road traffic accident. *Accident: Analysis and Prevention*, **43**, 471–7.

Cole, D. C., Mondloch, M. V., Hogg-Johnson, S., and the Early Claimant Cohort Prognostic Modelling Group. (2002) Listening to injured workers: How recovery expectations predict outcomes--a prospective study. *Canadian Medical Association Journal*, **166**, 749–54.

Cote, P., Hogg-Johnson, S., Cassidy, J. D., Carroll, L., and Frank, J. W. (2001) The association between neck pain intensity, physical functioning, depressive symptomatology and time-to-claim-closure after whiplash. *Journal of Clinical Epidemiology*, **54**, 275–86.

Crook, J., Milner, R., Schultz, I. Z., and Stringer, B. (2002) Determinants of occupational disability following a low back injury: A critical review of the literature. *Journal of Occupational Rehabilitation*, **12**, 277–95.

Currie, S. R., and Wang, J. L. (2004) Chronic back pain and major depression in the general Canadian population. *Pain*, **107**, 54–60.

da Silva, T., Macaskill, P., Mills, K., Maher, C., Williams, C., Lin, C. and Hancock. M. J. (2017) Predicting recovery in patients with acute low back pain: A clinical prediction model. *European Journal of Pain*, **21**, 716–26.

DeGood, D. E., and Kiernan, B. (1996) Perception of fault in patients with chronic pain. *Pain*, **64**, 153–9.

Dionne, C. E., Bourbonnais, R., Fremont, P. Rossignol, M., Stock, R., Nouwen, A., et al. (2006) Determinants of 'return to work in good health' among workers with back pain who consult in primary care settings: A 2-year prospective study. *European Spine Journal*, **16**, 641–55.

Du Bois, M., and Donceel, P. (2008) A screening questionnaire to predict no return to work within 3 months for low back pain claimants. *European Spine Journal*, **17**, 380–5.

Edwards, R. R., Dworkin, R. H., Sullivan, M. D., Turk, D. C., and Wasan, A. D. (2016) The role of psychosocial processes in the development and maintenance of chronic pain. *The Journal of Pain*, **17**, T70–92.

Elphinston, R. A., Thibault, P., Carriere, J. S., Rainville, P., and Sullivan, M.J. L. (2018) Cross-sectional and prospective correlates of recovery expectancies in the rehabilitation of whiplash injury. *Clinical Journal of Pain*, **34**, 306–12.

Ezenwa, M. O., Molokie, R. E., Wilkie, D. J., Suarez, M. L., and Yao, Y. (2014) Perceived injustice predicts stress and pain in adults with sickle cell disease. *Pain Management Nursing*, **16**, 294–306.

Ferrari, R., and Russell, A. S. (2014) Perceived injustice in fibromyalgia and rheumatoid arthritis. *Clinical Rheumatology*, **3**, 1501–7.

Fishbain, D. A., Pulikal, A., Lewis, J. E., and Gao, J. (2017) Chronic pain types differ in their reported prevalence of post-traumatic stress disorder (PTSD) and there is consistent evidence that chronic pain is associated with PTSD: An evidence-based structured systematic review. *Pain Medicine*, **18**, 711–35.

Fishbein, M., and Ajzen, I. (1975) *Belief, Attitude, Intention and behavior: An Introduction to Theory and Research*. Reading, MA: Addison-Wesley.

Friedrich, M. J. (2017) Depression is the leading cause of disability around the world. *JAMA*, **317**, 1517.

Fritz, J. M., George, S. Z., and Delitto, A. (2001) The role of fear-avoidance beliefs in acute low back pain: Relationships with current and future disability and work status. *Pain*, **94**, 7–15.

Gauthier, N., Sullivan, M. J., Adams, H., Stanish, W., and Thibault, P. (2006) Investigating risk factors for chronicity: The importance of distinguishing between return-to-work status and self-report measures of disability. *Journal of Occupational and Environmental Medicine*, **48**, 312–18.

Geisser, M. E., Roth, R. S., Bachman, J. E., and Eckert, T. A. (1996) The relationship between symptoms of post-traumatic stress disorder and pain, affective disturbance and disability among patients with accident and non-accident related pain. *Pain*, **66**, 207–14.

Goodin, B. R., McGuire, L., Allshouse, M., Stapleton, L., Haythornthwaite, J. A., Burns, N., et al. (2009) Associations between catastrophizing and endogenous pain-inhibitory processes: Sex differences. *The Journal of Pain*, **10**, 180–90.

Haefner, D. P., and Kirscht, J. P. (1970) Motivational and behavioral effects of modifying health beliefs. *Public Health Reports*, **85**, 478–84.

Hafer, C. L. and Begue, L. (2005) Experimental research on Just-World Theory: Problems, developments and future challenges. *Psychological Bulletin*, **131**, 128–67.

Hallegraeff, J. M., Krijnen, W. P., van der Schans, C. P. and de Greef, M. H. (2012) Expectations about recovery from acute non-specific low back pain predict absence from usual work due to chronic low back pain: A systematic review. *Journal of Physiotherapy*, **58**, 165–72.

Iles, R. A., Taylor, N. F., Davidson, M., and O'Halloran, P. D. (2012) Patient recovery expectations in non-chronic non-specific low back pain: A qualitative investigation. *Journal of Rehabilitation Medicine*, **44**, 781–7.

Iles, R. A., Davidson, M., and Taylor, N. F. (2008) Psychosocial predictors of failure to return to work in non-chronic non-specific low back pain: A systematic review. *Occupational and Environmental Medicine*, **65**, 507–17.

Jacobsen, P. B. and Butler, R. W. (1996) Relation of cognitive coping and catastrophizing to acute pain and analgesic use following breast cancer surgery. *Journal of Behavioral Medicine*, **19**, 17–29.

Janz, N. K. and Becker, M. H. (1984) The Health Belief Model: A decade later. *Health Education Quarterly*, **11**, 1–47.

Kirsch, I. (1985) Response expectancy as a determinant of experience and behavior. *The American Psychologist*, **40**, 1189–1202.

Kongsted, A., Bendix, T., Qerama, E., Kasch, H., Bach, F. W., Korsholm, L., and Jensen, T. S. (2008) Acute stress response and recovery after whiplash injuries. A one-year prospective study, *European Journal of Pain*, **12**, 455–63.

Kori, S. H., Miller, R. P., and Todd, D. D. (1990) Kinesiophobia: A new view of chronic pain behavior. *Pain Management*, **3**, 35–43.

Kozaric-Kovacic, D. (2009) Causes, diagnoses and treatment of post-traumatic stress disorder. *Acta Neuropsychiatrica*, **21** Suppl 2, 9.

Lackner, J. M., Carosella, A. M., and Feuerstein, M. (1996) Pain expectancies, pain, and functional self-efficacy expectancies as determinants of disability in patients with chronic low back disorders. *Journal of Consulting and Clinical Psychology*, **64**, 212–20.

Laisne, F., Lecomte, C., and Corbiere, M. (2013) Biopsychosocial determinants of work outcomes of workers with occupational injuries receiving compensation: A prospective study. *Work*, **44**, 117–32.

Lanier, D. C., and Stockton, P. (1988) Clinical predictors of outcome of acute episodes of low back pain. *Journal of Family Practice*, **27**, 483–9.

Leeuw, M., Goossens, M. E., Linton, S. J., Crombez, G., Boersma, K., and Vlaeyen, J. W. (2007) The fear-avoidance model of musculoskeletal pain: Current state of scientific evidence. *Journal of Behavioral Medicine*, **30**, 77–94.

Lotters, F., Franche, R. L., Hogg-Johnson, S., Burdorf, A. and Pole, J. D. (2006) The prognostic value of depressive symptoms, fear-avoidance, and self-efficacy for duration of lost-time benefits in workers with musculoskeletal disorders. *Occupational and Environmental Medicine*, **63**, 794–801.

Mankovsky, T., Lynch, M., Clark, A., Sawynok, J., and Sullivan, M. J. (2012) Pain catastrophizing predicts poor response to topical analgesics in patients with neuropathic pain. *Pain Research and Management*, **17**, 10–14.

Matthews, L. R. (2005) Work potential of road accident survivors with post-traumatic stress disorder. *Behaviour Research and Therapy*, **43**, 475–83.

Mayou, R. A., Ehlers, A., and Bryant, B. (2002) Posttraumatic stress disorder after motor vehicle accidents: 3-year follow-up of a prospective longitudinal study, *Behaviour Research and Therapy*, **40**, 665–75.

McParland, J. L., and Eccleston, C. (2013) 'It's not fair': Social justice appraisals in the context of chronic pain. *Current Directions in Psychological Science*, **22**, 484–9.

McParland, J. L., Eccleston, C., Osborn, M., and Hezseltine, L. (2011) It's not fair: An Interpretative Phenomenological Analysis of discourses of justice and fairness in chronic pain. *Health (London)*, **15**, 459–74.

McParland, J. L., and Whyte, A. (2008) A thematic analysis of attributions to others for the origins and ongoing nature of pain in community pain sufferers. *Psychology, Health and Medicine*, **13**, 610–20.

Moore, E., Thibault, P., Adams, A., and Sullivan, M. J. L. (2016) Catastrophizing and pain-related fear predict failure to maintain treatment gains following participation in a pain rehabilitation program. *Pain Reports*, 13, e567.

Nicholas, M. K. (2007) The pain self-efficacy questionnaire: Taking pain into account. *European Journal of Pain*, **11**, 153–63.

Overaas, C. K., Johansson, M. S., de Campos, T. F., Ferreira, M. L., Natvig, B., Mork, P. J., and Hartvigsen, J. (2017) Prevalence and pattern of co-occurring musculoskeletal pain and its association with back-related disability among people with persistent low back pain: Protocol for a systematic review and meta-analysis, *Systematic Reviews*, **6**, 258.

Pavlin, D. J., Sullivan, M. J., Freund, P. R., and Roesen, K. (2005) Catastrophizing: A risk factor for postsurgical pain. *The Clinical Journal of Pain*, **21**, 83–90.

Pelissier, C., Fort, E., Fontana, L., Charbotel, B., and Hours, M. (2017) Factors associated with non-return to work in the severely injured victims 3 years after a road accident: A prospective study. *Accident: Analysis and Prevention*, **106**, 411–19.

Peters, M. L., Sommer, M., de Rijke, J. M., Kessels, F., Heineman, E., Patijn, J., et al. (2007) Somatic and psychologic predictors of long-term unfavourable outcome after surgical intervention. *Annals of Surgery*, **245**, 487–94.

Pincus, T., Burton, A. K., Vogel, S., and Field, A. P. (2002) A systematic review of psychological factors as predictors of chronicity/disability in prospective cohorts of low back pain. *Spine*, **27**, E109–20.

Quartana, P. J., Campbell, C. M., and Edwards, R. R. (2009) Pain catastrophizing: A critical review. *Expert Review of Neurotherapeutics*, **9**, 745–58.

Richard, S., Dionne, C. E., and Nouwen, A. (2011) Self-efficacy and health locus of control: Relationship to occupational disability among workers with back pain. *Journal of Occupational Rehabilitation*, **21**, 421–30.

Rodero, B., Luciano J. V., Montero-Marin, J., Casanueva, B., Palacin, J. C., Gili, M., et al. (2012) Perceived injustice in fibromyalgia: Psychometric characteristics of the Injustice Experience Questionnaire and relationship with pain catastrophising and pain acceptance. *Journal of Psychosomatic Research*, **73**, 86–91.

Rush, A. J., Polatin, P., and Gatchel, R. J. (2000) Depression and chronic low back pain: Establishing priorities in treatment, *Spine*, **25**, 2566–71.

Sarda, J., Jr., Nicholas, M.K., Asghari, A., and Pimenta, C.A. (2009) The contribution of self-efficacy and depression to disability and work status in chronic pain patients: A comparison between Australian and Brazilian samples. *European Journal of Pain*, **13**, 189–95.

Schultz, I. Z., Crook, J. M., Berkowitz, J., Meloche, G. R., Milner, R. O., Zuberbier, A., and Meloche, W. (2002) Biopsychosocial multivariate predictive model of occupational low back disability. *Spine*, **27**, 2720–5.

Schutze, R., Rees, C., Smith, A., Slater, H., Campbell, J. M., and O'Sullivan, P. (2018) How can we best reduce pain catastrophizing in adults with chronic noncancer pain? A systematic review and meta-analysis. *The Journal of Pain*, **19**, 233–56.

Scott, W., and Sullivan, M. J. L. (2012) Perceived injustice moderates the relationship between pain and depressive symptoms among individuals with persistent musculoskeletal pain. *Pain Research and Management*, **17**, 335–40.

Scott, W., Trost, Z., Milioto, M., and Sullivan, M. J. L. (2015) Barriers to change in depressive symptoms following multidisciplinary rehabilitation for whiplash: The role of perceived injustice. *Clinical Journal of Pain*, **31**, 145–51.

Scott, W., Trost, Z., Milioto, M., and Sullivan, M. J. L. (2013) Further validation of a measure of injury-related injustice perceptions to identify risk for occupational disability: A prospective study of individuals with whiplash injury. *Journal of Occupational Rehabilitation*, **23**, 557–65.

Scott, W., Wideman, T. H., and Sullivan, M. J. (2014) Clinically meaningful scores on pain catastrophizing before and after multidisciplinary rehabilitation: A prospective study of individuals with subacute pain after whiplash injury. *The Clinical Journal of Pain*, **30**, 183–90.

Smith, A. D., Jull, G. A., Schneider, G. M., Frizzell, B., Hooper, R. A. and Sterling, M. M. (2016) Low pain catastrophization and disability predict successful outcome to radiofrequency neurotomy in individuals with chronic whiplash. *Pain Practice*, **16**, 311–19.

Smith, A. D., Jull, G., Schneider, G., Frizzell, B., Hooper, R. A., and Sterling, M. (2013) A comparison of physical and psychological features of responders and non-responders to cervical facet blocks in chronic whiplash. *BMC Musculoskeletal Disorders*, **14**, 313.

Sobin, C., and Sackeim, H. A. (1997) Psychomotor symptoms of depression. *American Journal of Psychiatry*, **154**, 4–17.

Sullivan, M. J., Stanish, W., Sullivan, M. E., and Tripp, D. (2002) Differential predictors of pain and disability in patients with whiplash injuries. *Pain Research and Management*, **7**, 68–74.

Sullivan, M. J. L. (2003) Emerging trends in secondary prevention of pain-related disability. *The Clinical Journal of Pain*, **19**, 77–9.

Sullivan, M. J. L., Adams, A., and Ellis, T. (2012) Targeting catastrophic thinking to promote return to work in individuals with fibromyalgia. *Journal of Cognitive Psychotherapy*, **26**, 130–42.

Sullivan, M. J. L., and Adams, H. (2010) Psychosocial treatment techniques to augment the impact of physiotherapy interventions for low back pain. *Physiotherapy Canada*, **62**, 180–9.

Sullivan, M. J. L., Adams, H., Horan, S., Maher, D., Boland, D., and Gross, R. (2008) The role of perceived injustice in the experience of chronic pain and disability: Scale development and validation. *Journal of Occupational Rehabilitation*, **18**, 249–61.

Sullivan, M. J. L., Adams, H., Martel, M. O., Scott, W., and Wideman, T. (2011) Catastrophizing and perceived injustice: Risk factors for the transition to chronicity after whiplash injury. *Spine*, **36**, S244–9.

Sullivan, M. J. L., Adams, H., Rhodenizer, T., and Stanish, W. D. (2006) A psychosocial risk factor--targeted intervention for the prevention of chronic pain and disability following whiplash injury. *Physical Therapy*, **86**, 8–18.

Sullivan, M. J. L., Adams, H., Thibault, P., Corbiere, M., and Stanish, W. D. (2006) Initial depression severity and the trajectory of recovery following cognitive-behavioral intervention for work disability. *Journal of Occupational Rehabilitation*, **16**, 63–74.

Sullivan, M. J. L., Feuerstein, M., Gatchel, R., Linton, S. J., and Pransky, G. (2005) Integrating psychosocial and behavioral interventions to achieve optimal rehabilitation outcomes. *Journal of Occupational Rehabilitation*, **15**, 475–89.

Sullivan, M. J. L., and Hyman, M. (2014) Return to work as a treatment objective for patients with chronic pain? *Journal of Pain and Relief*, **3**, 1–3.

Sullivan, M. J. L., and Stanish, W. D. (2003) Psychologically-based occupational rehabilitation: The Pain-Disability Prevention Program. *The Clinical Journal of Pain*, **19**, 97–104.

Sullivan, M. J. L., Stanish, W., Waite, H., Sullivan, M., and Tripp, D. A. (1998) Catastrophizing, pain, and disability in patients with soft-tissue injuries. *Pain*, **77**, 253–60.

Sullivan, M. J. L., Thibault, P., Simmonds, M.J., Milioto, M., Cantin, A. P., and Velly, A. M. (2009) Pain, perceived injustice and the persistence of post-traumatic stress symptoms during the course of rehabilitation for whiplash injuries. *Pain*, **145**, 325–31.

Sullivan, M. J. L., Thorn, B., Haythornthwaite, J. A., Keefe, F., Martin, M., Bradley, L. A., and Lefebvre, J. C. (2001) Theoretical perspectives on the relation between catastrophizing and pain. *The Clinical Journal of Pain*, 17, 52–64.

Sullivan, M. J. L., Ward, L. C., Tripp, D., French, D. J., Adams, H., and Stanish, W. D. (2005) Secondary prevention of work disability: Community-based psychosocial intervention for musculoskeletal disorders. *Journal of Occupational Rehabilitation*, 15, 377–92.

Sullivan, M. J. L., Yakobov, E., Scott, W., and Tait, R. C. (2014) Perceived injustice and adverse recovery outcomes. *Psychological Injury and Law*, 7, 325–34.

Sullivan, M. J. L., Reesor, K., Mikail, S., and Fisher, R. (1992) The treatment of depression in chronic low back pain: Review and recommendations. *Pain*, 50, 5–13.

Thibault, P., Loisel, P., Durand, M. J., Catchlove, R., and Sullivan, M. J. L. (2008) Psychological predictors of pain expression and activity intolerance in chronic pain patients. *Pain*, 139, 47–54.

Trost, Z., Strachan, E., Sullivan, M., Vervoort,T., Avery, A. R., and Afari, N. (2015) Heritability of pain catastrophizing and associations with experimental pain outcomes: A twin study. *Pain*, 156, 514–20.

Turk, D. C. (2002) A diathesis-stress model of chronic pain and disability. *Pain Research and Management*, 7, 9–19.

Turk, D. C. (1996) Biopsychosocial perspective on chronic pain. In: Gatchel, R. J., and Turk, D. C. (eds.) *Psychological Approaches to Pain Management*. New York: Guilford, 3–29.

Turk, D. C., and Okifuji, A. (2002) Psychological factors in chronic pain: Evolution and revolution. *Journal of Consulting and Clinical Psychology*, 70, 678–90.

Turner, J. A., Franklin, G., Fulton-Kehoe, D., Sheppard, L., Wickizer, T. M., Wu, R. et al. (2006) Worker recovery expectations and fear-avoidance predict work disability in a population-based workers' compensation back pain sample, *Spine*, 31, 682–9.

Vargas-Prada, S., and Coggon, D. (2015) Psychological and psychosocial determinants of musculoskeletal pain and associated disability, *Best Practice and Research. Clinical Rheumatology*, 29, 374–90.

Verbunt, J. A., Sieben, J., Vlaeyen, J. W., Portegijs, P., and Andre Knottnerus, J. (2008) A new episode of low back pain: Who relies on bed rest? *European Journal of Pain*, 12, 508–16.

Verkerk, K., Luijsterburg, P. A., Miedema, H. S., Pool-Goudzwaard, A., and Koes, B. W. (2012) Prognostic factors for recovery in chronic nonspecific low back pain: A systematic review. *Physical Therapy*, 92, 1093–108.

Vlaeyen, J. W., de Jong, J., Geilen, M., Heuts, P. H., and van Breukelen, G. (2001) Graded exposure in vivo in the treatment of pain-related fear: A replicated single-case experimental design in four patients with chronic low back pain. *Behaviour Research and Therapy*, 39, 151–66.

Vlaeyen, J. W., and Linton, S. J. (2000) Fear-avoidance and its consequences in chronic musculoskeletal pain: A state of the art. *Pain*, 85, 317–32.

Vowles, K. E., Gross, R. T., and Sorrell, J. T. (2004) Predicting work status following interdisciplinary treatment for chronic pain. *European Journal of Pain*, 8, 351–8.

Waddell, G., Newton, M., Henderson, I., Somerville, D., and Main, C. J. (1993) A Fear-Avoidance Beliefs Questionnaire (FABQ) and their role of fear-avoidance beliefs in chronic low back pain and disability. *Pain*, 52, 157–68.

Wenzel, H. G., Haug, T. T., Mykletun, A., and Dahl, A. A. (2002) A population study of anxiety and depression among persons who report whiplash traumas. *Journal of Psychosomatic Research*, 53, 831–5.

Wideman, T. H., and Sullivan, M. J. (2011a) Differential predictors of the long-term levels of pain intensity, work disability, healthcare use, and medication use in a sample of workers' compensation claimants. *Pain*, **152**, 376–83.

Wideman, T. H., and Sullivan, M. J. L. (2011b) Reducing catastrophic thinking associated with pain. *Pain Management*, **1**, 249–56.

Yakobov, E., Scott, W., Stanish, W., Dunbar, M., Richardson, G., and Sullivan, M. J. L. (2014) The role of perceived injustice in the prediction of pain and function following total knee arthroplasty. *Pain*, **155**, 2040–6.

Yakobov, E., Suso-Ribera, C., Vrinceanu, T., Adams, H., and Sullivan, M. J. L. (2019) Trait perceived injustice is associated with pain intensity and pain behaviour in participants undergoing an experimental pain induction procedure. *Journal of Pain,* **20**, 592–9.

Chapter 10

Managing pain-related limitations in the workplace: The role of the employer

Chris J. Main and William S. Shaw

Introduction

The main focus of this chapter is on pain-related work limitations (PWL),[§] and in particular on the role of the employer and the challenges of implementing change in an occupational environment often focused sharply on profit and the avoidance of litigation. It will be argued that full and appropriate engagement in a healthy and motivated workforce is in everyone's interests, although changes in the types of work, in working conditions and in increasingly diverse work practices, represent real challenges in the design of interventions and their implementation in practice.

In this chapter we begin with a description and attempted quantification of the burden of PWL. We then offer a review of the major organizational processes, the influence of management structures and prognostic factors before considering workplace interventions, and the influence of health/social policy. We conclude with a series of recommendations for an integrated approach to the management of PWL.

The burden of PWL

Costs

The single greatest cause globally of YLDs (Years Living with Disability) is chronic low back pain, with an increase of 61% since 1990, with the main four chronic pain conditions accounting for 20.8% of all YLDs globally in 2013 (Vos et al., 2016); and a massive increase in the prevalence of opioid use disorders since 1990. According to Rice et al., (2016), the burden associated with chronic pain is in many cases increasing, due in part to powerful demographic forces such as the aging of populations in the developed countries and increased survival into middle and old age in the developing

---

[§] In this chapter the term 'Pain Related Work Limitations' (PWL) and 'Health Related Work Limitations' (HWL) often will be used in preference to the term 'work disability' which is used slightly differently in the USA and Europe for which the favoured metric tends to be economic rather than performance deficit.

countries. Work disability is thus a huge burden, from industrialized societies at one end down to the individual person living with the disability (Shaw et al., 2016).

The impact of pain on work

Treatment, rehabilitation and primary prevention have been addressed primarily in terms of biomechanics and ergonomics but pain can also have a significant effect on cognitive function, mood, and fatigue, with concomitant changes in communication and social interactions, all of which can be additional obstacles to re-integration into work.

Work can be a source of distress for some, worsening mental health conditions (OECD, 2015). A range of factors including low quality jobs, poor leaders, and psychosocial stress at work can create difficult psychosocial conditions for workers, and even set off specific mental health conditions (Stansfeld and Candy, 2006). An unhealthy and unhappy workforce is costly in terms of sickness absence, presenteeism, and reduced productivity.

Almost 20% of workers with back pain take some absence over a period of 6 months or longer, with return to work (RTW) rates of 68% at up to 1 month, 85% at 1–6 months, and 93% at 6 months' follow-up (Wynne Jones et al., 2014).

The impact on health of the modern working environment

Differences in working conditions and practice are evident in the nature and organization of work, employee rights, reporting arrangements, protection in relation to health-related work limitations (HWL), and employer support. In the management of PWL there are a wide range of potential barriers to be overcome (Kristman et al., 2016). However, there are also clear financial and psychosocial benefits of health and well-being to the worker. The benefit of efficacious management of PWL to employers includes: increased productivity; lower rates of early retirement due to ill health; reduced absenteeism and quick return to work after illness; fewer workplace injuries; greater staff retention and engaged employees; reduced costs to train new staff; improvements in communications; and a more positive corporate image (Kristman et al., 2016).

Impact of chronic health conditions and an ageing workforce

The prevalence of chronic health conditions in the workforce is increasing (Fried et al., 2012). It is estimated that by 2020, at least 35% of the workforce in many countries will be aged 55 or more and a significant proportion can be expected to suffer from HWL in general and PWL in particular (Leijten et al., 2014). Particular issues that older workers with chronic health conditions can face in the workplace include tiredness, emotional exhaustion, varying levels of help from other workers and managers, and challenges in modifying their roles at work (Varekamp et al., 2008) and they may have very different work disability considerations, for example they may be close to retirement or already working within post-retirement jobs or careers. They may have less economic pressure or personal need to return to work after a period of disability and may prefer instead to consider alternative forms of occupation. Alternatively, older workers may prefer to remain at work to accrue further income and enjoy the social engagement that work can bring.

When an injury occurs, older workers often suffer more serious injuries than their younger counterparts, take longer to come back to work, work claims are more costly, and they are more likely to leave the workplace again having attempted to return. As highlighted by Pransky et al. (2016), 'although some work disability problems observed in aging workers are primarily related to health, other factors—such as competing retirement options, career status, likelihood of accommodations and mobility in the workforce—are specific to age group and career stage, and can interact with health' (Berecki-Gisolf et al., 2012). Further, Pransky et al. (2016) note that 'the growth of an aging workforce has heightened employer concerns about the ability of older workers to remain at work given their higher rate of medical illness, and increased risk for work disability'.

The influence of organizational processes

Clinical and occupational health interventions to be focused at the level of the individual worker typically do not require consideration at an organizational level, but workplace-centred interventions traditionally are directed at the workforce as a whole (although the distinction is not absolute) and involve consideration of organizational processes.

The challenge of implementation

The success of interventions for PWL is dependent not only on the intervention per se but on its implementation (Main et al., 2016), which is often dependent on the determinants of behaviour change, many of which are contextual in nature. With PWL, the principal context is the individual's working environment which of course may be populated by a range of individuals, including managers, supervisors, and working colleagues. However challenging this may appear, the workplace can offer a range of possibilities for workplace-based interventions.

Organizational culture and climate

*Organizational culture has been defined as the *shared values, assumptions, and beliefs* that are communicated in the behaviours that the organization uses to overcome prior problems, thereby validating the importance of these actions (Schneider et al., 2013) and is often discussed in terms of three layers:

---

* Section 'Organization culture and climate' adapted under the terms of the Creative Commons Attribution 4.0 International License, http://creativecommons.org/licenses/by/4.0/ from Main C.J. *et al.* (2016). Implementation science and employer disability practices: embedding implementation factors in research designs. *J Occup Rehabil.* 26(4):448–464. Copyright © The Author(s) 2016. https://doi.org/10.1007/s10926-016-9677-7.

1. Artefacts (e.g. how people dress, how the space is arranged, etc.), but the meaning of which may vary from organization to organization;

2. Espoused values (i.e. as declared by the organizational members and management);

3. Underlying assumptions (typically shared throughout the organization and that drive how employees interact and behave, although not always explicitly acknowledged).

Thus, organizational culture is generally quite broad, encompassing all of these layers and almost all aspects of organizational life (Dodek et al., 2010).

Organizational climate has been defined as the shared perception of the work environment including the policies, practices, and procedures that guide the expected, supported, and rewarded behaviours (Ehrhart et al., 2014).

In recent years, there has been a growing interest further in the concept of implementation climate as an integrative framework linking the organization and the worker (Damshroder et al., 2009) and which captures specifically the expectations, support, and rewards associated with implementation. Multiple measures have been developed (Jacobs et al., 2014). Unfortunately, while these factors may have explanatory utility, to date, outcomes of attempts to change organizational culture in health care, have been disappointing (Curry et al., 2015), but the constructs do provide a framework for approaching possible organizational interventions and are commonly included in models of organizational change.

Organizational readiness to change

*Strategies that involve assessment, intervention, and support for implementation at multiple organizational levels should have a greater likelihood of success (Aarons et al., (2015). Organizational readiness to change (Weiner, 2009) seems to be of particular importance (Jones et al., 2005) in terms of organizational members' change commitment and efficacy in implementing change (Weiner et al., 2008). However, there may be significant differences in the perception of roles and tasks between stakeholders (Franche et al., 2005) and potential barriers should be identified and, if possible, addressed prior to implementation of the intervention.

The influence of management structures

The role of the employer

The typical role of the employer has expanded from being a manufacturer/provider of goods and a purchaser of labour, to making reasonable allowance in terms of ergonomic and biomechanical adjustments, sometimes accompanied by a phased return-to-work plan after sickness absence or injury. These developments have

---

* Section 'Organizational readiness to change' adapted under the terms of the Creative Commons Attribution 4.0 International License, http://creativecommons.org/licenses/by/ 4.0/ from Main C. J. et al. (2016). Implementation science and employer disability practices: embedding implementation factors in research designs. *J Occup Rehabil*. 26(4):448–464. Copyright © The Author(s) 2016. https://doi.org/10.1007/s10926-016-9677-7.

highlighted the central importance of the relationship of the employee with their supervisor, manager, and colleagues; and energized a move from the traditional adversarial stance which characterized industrial relations to mutual engagement of the various stakeholders in collaborative initiatives focused on common, agreed, and negotiated goals. Furthermore, there has been a particular research focus on the influence of leadership and the nature of line management (Boardman and Lyon, 2006).

Transformational leadership (Eisenbeiss et al., 2008) has been linked to organizational innovation across a group of studies, often via its impact on the organizational environment. Four dimensions of implementation leadership have been identified: "knowledgeable leadership, supportive leadership, proactive leadership, and perseverant leadership" (Main et al., 2016, p. 455; see also, Aarons et al, 2014).

Middle managers also have an important role to play, especially in knowledge-intensive businesses. They may have a larger impact on organizational performance than nearly any other part of an organization, and much more than that of individual creative team members (Wharton Business School, 2010). The best managers are able to work closely with the innovators to turn their ideas into realistic project plans, and they are effective at motivating the team and facilitating collective creativity.

Although relatively few studies have focused on the relationship between line managers' behaviours and the outcomes of occupational health interventions, it has been shown not only that line managers' attitudes and actions positively predict changes in both self-rated health and work ability, but also that the influence of transformational leadership is mediated through line managers' attitudes and actions towards the intervention (Lundmark et al., 2017).

Workplace prognostic factors

As outlined in Main and Shaw (2016), 'psychosocial factors such as job autonomy, job demands, and emotionally demanding work are more strongly associated with low performance at work than with sickness absence' (see also Böckerman and Laukkanen, 2010). Occupational factors in back disability include physical and psychological demands, as well as social/managerial factors. Worker perceptions and beliefs and perceptions of work and working conditions have been identified as potential obstacles to recovery/optimal function (Shaw et al., 2009). For some purposes it is helpful to distinguish between *worker-centred* interventions (such as provided by clinical services and occupational health (frequently outsourced), and *workplace-centred* interventions (Sullivan et al., 2005) which affect groups of workers or the entire workforce.

Nicholas et al. (2011), after an evidence-based review, concluded that if risk factors we can modify are targeted directly rather than indiscriminately, good outcomes may be attained. Schultz et al. (2016) discussed how in one of the few studies which directly compared prognostic factors for RTW, 32% of the variance in RTW was explained, using a combination of Yellow and Blue Flags: 'Workers with acute low back pain at highest risk for delayed RTW: (1) expected to stay on sick leave for more

---

Box 10.1 Levers of intervention in the workplace

- At the worker level: *individual stress management and methods to include personal control; focus on demands of greatest concern to the individual*
- At the workforce level: *include affected co-workers in RTW strategy; provide general workforce re-education and improve awareness*
- At the supervisor level: *adapt medical restrictions to facilitate job modifications and accommodations; train for improved supportive communication*
- At the managerial level: *develop a clear set of policies and apply consistently; include disability prevention as part of wider focus on health and wellness.*

Adapted under the Attribution 4.0 International (CC BY 4.0), https://creativecommons.org/licenses/by/4.0/ from Kristman V. L. et al. Researching Complex and Multi-Level Workplace Factors Affecting Disability and Prolonged Sickness Absence. *J Occup Rehabil.* 26 (4): 399–416. Copyright © 2016 The Author(s). https://doi.org/10.1007/s10926-016-9660-3.

---

than 10 days, (2) were being treated by a general practitioner or medical specialist, (3) were unable to appear at the occupational physician's office; and (4) had a 10.8 times higher risk for delayed RTW. Similarly, the high- risk workers for lasting RTW as well as factors 1 and 2 for RTW, also reported job stress as a cause of sick leave' (Steenstra et al., 2005).

Workplace interventions

A wide range of different types of workplace interventions are reported, but it has been recommended that distinctions are made between four specific levels of intervention (the individual worker, the supervisor, the manager, and the workplace), each associated with a different focus on disability and types of intervention strategy (Kristman et al., 2016) (see Box 10.1).

However, research into workers with chronic illness who are successful at work, despite enduring ill health, advocate new approaches that may help, and illustrate that intervention may function across levels. For example, employees living with chronic pain reported that altering work routines and activities, decreasing pain symptoms, using cognitive techniques, and communicating well about pain were key. Six main themes were reported: knowing your work setting, talking about pain, being prepared for a bad day, thoughts and emotions, keeping moving, and finding leeway (Tveito et al., 2010). Research into workers with ongoing medical conditions show that supervisor support and being able to modify work are critical issues (Munir et al., 2009), although interestingly, line managers viewed employer/employee cooperation as most important, yet human resource managers paid more attention to the importance of organizational culture and policy in relation to working with ongoing ill-health conditions (Haafkens et al., 2011).

The focus of workplace policies

*Workplace policies and programmes typically struggle with intermittent work absence that can occur because of chronic illnesses, and generally focus on the administrative complexities of managing entitlements such as sick leave benefits, rather than the opportunity for coordinating medical care and workplace accommodation. However, the functional impacts of chronic illness can vary greatly over time, and so an employee-driven approach may offer a more flexible and responsive solution than requesting a formal accommodation each time there is a change in health and functional ability, as long as the accommodations are reasonable for both employer and employee.

Self-management and supervisor support

†Work accommodations are an essential component of work disability prevention in workers with chronic illness (Boot et al., 2013) and workplaces are experimenting with a bottom-up non-medical strategy for workplace accommodations. In these models, employees and their supervisors have the primary responsibility for figuring out accommodations; and the grey literature reports cite greatly improved work absence outcomes (Scott-Parker, 2014). Recently, interventions have attempted to enhance self-management and supervisor support in the workplace. Results so far have indicated improved self-efficacy for staying at work, but no significant impact on RTW or work retention (Hutting et al., 2015). However provision of reassurance, facilitating accommodations, and problem-solving, have been successful in decreasing work absence (Werner et al., 2007).

The need for a redirection of effort in the management of PWL

While the scientific literature is focused on facilitating improved coping and reducing discomforts for individual workers, the employer-directed grey literature is focused on making group-level changes to policies and procedures. Future research might better target employer practices by tying interventions to positive workplace influences and determinants, by developing more participatory interventions and research designs, and by designing interventions that address factors of organizational change

---

and organizational readiness. The beliefs and values of senior managers would seem to be critical factors in facilitating changes in such disability management practices. (Williams-Whitt et al., 2016)

Influence of health/social policy on the management of PWL

Recognition of fundamental changes in the nature of work and working conditions has necessitated re-examination of the nature and management of health-related work compromise (HWL), resulting in a comprehensive evidence review (Waddell et al., 2006), and the influential Carol Black Report (Black, 2008) which identified a key role for the workplace in promoting health and well-being. Subsequently, the UK Government in its recent 10-year plan (DOH, 2017) attempted to address the problem of HWL (work disability) by joining up activity across three key settings—the welfare system, the workplace, and the health-care system, with the aspiration of providing support for those who need it, whatever their health conditions or disability; although the strategy has not received unconditional support (Shakespeare et al., 2016).

The report *inter alia* identifies a crucial role for managers and supervisors in creating healthy and inclusive workplaces, and in creating opportunities for people who need a more flexible approach. It also recognizes the need for health-care professionals to be ready to talk about health barriers to work; to provide timely access to appropriate treatments; to develop effective occupational health services, within but also beyond the NHS, giving access for everyone including small businesses and the self-employed; and to develop a focus on prevention and early intervention.

A broadening of focus from sickness to wellness

Implicit in the new strategy has been 'consideration of well-being, not only as an outcome of intervention but also as a potential mediator of improved adjustment and performance and requiring consideration both of the positive and the negative aspects of the work environment' (Tetrick et al., 2012).

Weiner et al. (2009) has proposed an organizational theoretical model to better understand the complex pathways to the success of worksite wellness programs. Key features of this model include: organizational readiness to change, extant and new policies and practices, a managerial and employee climate relevant to the implementation, effectiveness of the implementation, and fit with the culture and values of the workplace.

In an early review of 110 worksite-based wellness interventions, Harden et al. (1999) concluded that key factors related to success included 'visible and enthusiastic support for, and involvement in, the intervention from top management; involvement of employees at all organizational levels in the planning, implementation and activities of the intervention; and tailoring for the characteristics and needs of the recipients' (p. 546). A more recent review (McCoy et al., 2014) of studies of workplace factors related to the success of wellness programs in small workplaces concluded that managerial support, a culture of health, and organizational policy changes were key organizational factors, in addition to adequate facilities, budget, and expertise.

However, the overall effect of workplace health promotion interventions appears to be small, is partly determined by intervention characteristics, and high-quality RCTs report lower effect sizes (Rongen et al., 2013). This may be a consequence in part of the difficulty in implementing change. After Martins (2011), and as previously highlighted in Main et al. (2016), we highlight five key threats to the success of organizational change efforts: '(a) lack of an adequate framework for implementing organizational change; (b) failure to accurately identify the problem; (c) inaccurate diagnosis of the problem and its root causes; (d) lack of fidelity in the implementation of a planned intervention; and (e) inadequate measurement of the resulting effect or insufficient time given' (p. 456).

It seems, therefore, that conclusions about workplace interventions drawn from health promotion/wellness literature, while encouraging, should be treated with some caution.

The implementation of policy recommendations

Culture, leadership, and people management have been identified as core underpinnings of engagement but engagement of employers (the way in which the business care is articulated and communicated) is a major challenge (Suff and Miller, 2016). They translated five behaviourally focused themes (competencies) into 54 behavioural indicators which could be assessed as a basis for action. They recognized that in order to manage a sustainable engagement framework, there was a need for clear, open, and fair communication; provision of advice and guidance; the building of teams in sustained relationships; and support for employee development. They also advocated: a concerted focus on advancing the qualitative aspects of jobs and working lives; with clear paths to career progression; access to flexible working; improved line management and HR capability; and reduction in excessive workload and stress with the championing of mental health and overall well-being.

All well and good, but aspirational rather operational. Some recommendations about how this might be undertaken are presented below.

Recent developments

*The establishment of a new cross-department Work and Health Unit by the UK government has been accompanied by new policy recommendations (Taylor et al., 2017) which signal a move beyond health and well-being to a complete reconsideration of work practices, and bring the role of the employer, and their relationships with employees, into sharp focus. A key feature in this new approach is the engagement

---

of all interested stakeholders as opposed to exclusive outsourcing to health-care personnel in identifying and tackling the determinants of behaviour change in interventions at various levels, and improving outcomes as measured by relevant and agreed metrics. The suggested 'deconstruction' of the challenge of work disability into a series of linked problems requires the inclusion of both worker-centred and workplace-centred initiatives into the re-integration process.

This development sits well with the conclusions of a recent special issue on employer practices (Main and Shaw, 2016) which *inter alia* recommended the re-conceptualization of work disability as a problem of sustained re-integration into work. This term can encompass both traditional perspectives on work disability and contextual analyses of the nature of the work environment; and as a potential determinant of successful re-integration into work. Before interventions are introduced, a re-engagement analysis should be conducted. This analysis should commence with consideration of possible interventions (Williams-Whitt et al., 2016); accounting for the characteristics of the targeted population (Pransky et al., 2016); factoring in differences in the type of work and working conditions (Ekberg et al., 2016); and proceeding with identification of all stakeholders and maximizing their involvement.

Developments in the management of PWL

Two further specific developments in the management of PWL merit mention. First, a proposal has been mooted for development of an intervention toolbox to '(1) minimise the occurrence of work-relevant common health problems (CHPs) and (2) reduce avoidable sickness absence, healthcare use and long-term disability for CHP complaints that inevitably occur in the workplace' (Kendall et al., 2015, p. v). Although directed at common health problems the proposal is clearly relevant to PWL. The primary intent is to enable people to continue 'work participation, measured by ability to stay at work or return speedily after absence, thus sustaining productive activity. The conceptual model spans three key areas: good work; good jobs; and supportive workplaces' (Kendall et al., 2015, p. vi) (see Box 10.2).

Second, a new type of service has been proposed (Christian et al., 2016). It is dedicated to responding rapidly to new health-related work absence among working people due to potentially disabling conditions by attending to the worker's basic needs and concerns (Shaw et al., 2013) and the medical, functional restoration, and occupational aspects of the situation are addressed in a coordinated fashion (Wickizer et al., 2011). The modest set of simple services is characterized by an immediate, systematic, pro-active, integrated, and multidimensional approach to both clinical and occupational concerns. However, as with the intervention toolbox proposal, the key challenge is likely to be the implementation rather than the content of the intervention/service.

Remaining challenges

The challenges of an ageing workforce have already been highlighted, but there are two further major challenges which perhaps should be recognized.

Box 10.2 Conceptual model

Good work includes the provision of good jobs for when people are well, and supportive workplaces for when they are ill or injured.

Good jobs **are characterized by:** balanced demands and a safe work environment; effective and helpful line management; working practices and feedback that lead workers to feel they are valued and respected members of staff. The jobs are also characterized by opportunities to use and develop skills; endorsement and opportunities for workers to solve their own problems; encouragement to help workers make their own work better; and, opportunities for social interaction.

Supportive workplaces **are characterized by:** commitment from senior management; early provision of factual information and advice; fostering early reporting of work-relevant health problems; keeping in touch; adopting a can-do approach; engaging the person in identifying obstacles to work participation and making a work plan; assessing the job and offering temporary modified work if needed (just to ease the path to usual work); liaising with health-care practitioners if necessary (using a confidentiality waiver); allowing graduated return to work plans; and monitoring progress so the plan can be appropriately revised if there are any setbacks.

Adapted from Kendall N. et al. *Developing an intervention toolbox for common health problems in the workplace*. Health and Safety Executive. © Crown Copyright 2015. Available from http://www.hse.gov.uk/research/rrhtm/rr1053.htm. Contains public sector information licensed under the Open Government Licence v3.0.

Fostering inclusion and managing diversity

The creation of a climate of inclusion (Shore et al., 2010) requires fairness in implementation of employment practices, integration of differences, and inclusion in decision making (Nishii, 2013) which promote employees' needs for both belongingness and uniqueness being satisfied. Evidence for success in the establishment of inclusiveness is as yet limited but suggests the need for new types of partnership built on a stronger foundation of shared understanding and aspiration.

Dealing with a continually changing working environment

Most workplace research carried out on disability prevention and RTW has focused on 'conventional' workplaces, often large organizations which have been the 'gold standard' but work is often characterized by on-demand employment offering limited or no societal protection, (Ekberg et al., 2016). Groups particularly vulnerable to insecure work arrangements include the lower-educated, immigrants, chronically ill, and individuals with disabilities. Those experiencing 'precarious employment arrangements and non-standard working-times... are more likely to report higher exposure to psychosocial workplace risks, higher levels of behavioural health disorders, such as

Box 10.3 Recommendations

1. The challenge of HWL in general and PWL in particular (work disability) should be re-conceptualized as a problem of *sustained reintegration into work*; a term which can complement traditional perspectives on work disability with a contextual analysis of the nature of the workplace as a potential determinant of successful reintegration into work. This necessitates the involvement of all interested parties rather than exclusive outsourcing to healthcare personnel.

2. Such a conceptualization invites consideration of the determinants of behaviour change at multiple levels and places the process of implementation at the centre of the stage. In this analysis we need to identify the behavioural changes required by both the organization and the 'injured' worker and construct a multi-faceted intervention.

3. We should attempt to incorporate influences on implementation as part of the design of the intervention, rather than as confounders of treatment outcome (perhaps requiring a deconstructing of the challenge of work disability into a series of linked problems which need to be addressed).

4. The inclusion of both worker-centred and workplace-centred initiatives into the reintegration process, may require a fundamental change in organization culture (including a focus on work retention, as a means of preventing unnecessary disability).

5. We recommend a broader concept of relevant science and research methods, informed by organizational psychology, organizational development and social psychology, although the marked diversity in workplaces, workforces, and in the specifics of pain-associated work compromise, remain major challenges.

6. Prior to introducing interventions we advocate a *re-engagement analysis* beginning with consideration of possible interventions; taking into account the characteristics of the targeted population; factoring in differences in the type of work and working conditions; proceeding with identification of all stakeholders, applying recent advances in implementation science as to how the intervention might be implemented, and taking into account the need for careful and appropriate measurement at every stage of the process.

7. Finally, in so doing, we need to accommodate the difference in perspective between clinical/organizational scientists and employers in terms of overall objectives, agreed outcomes, and ensure full engagement with the implementation process.

depression, anxiety, and sleep problems, higher levels of work absenteeism and higher 'presenteeism,' and related physical and psychosocial risks' (Ekberg et al., 2016).

It would seem that investment is required into capturing the influence of such changes on both well-being and performance, but in order to do so, the sharing of information among all parties will require attention to the nature and effectiveness of communication across and between all levels of organizations.

Conclusions and recommendations

The long-standing aim of curing all forms of disability (whether via medical intervention or by developing biomechanically based ergonomic solutions) before a return to work no longer appears feasible and new solutions are needed to assist RTW and sustain work engagement, despite ongoing symptoms.

It seems apparent that the effectiveness of occupational interventions for PWL will probably not improve without paying proper attention to the context of where the intervention will occur and how we can facilitate its implementation.

Within the broad canvas of PWL and its management are many implications specifically for employers and we have commented on their role, above. We suggest they need to be central participants in the management of PWL rather than purchasers of out-sourced services.

There will always be a quest for a clinical cure for intermittent and chronic PWL, but in our view the challenge of PWL lies as much in the organizational environment as in the individual worker. We consider that the overarching task in PWL management is the facilitation of sustained behaviour change (at the level of both the worker and the organization) and our energies might be best deployed in identifying and tackling the determinants of behaviour change (see Box 10.3).

Acknowledgements

This chapter contains public sector information licensed under the Open Government Licence v3.0.

The authors would like to acknowledge gratefully, help from Kim Burton in signposting key material to us.

References

Aarons, G. A., Ehrhart, M. G., and Farahnak, L. R. (2014) The implementation leadership scale (ILS): Development of a brief measure of unit level implementation leadership. *Implementation Science*, **9**, 45.

Aarons, G. A., Ehrhart, M. G., Farahnak, L. R., and Hurlburt, M. S.(2015) Leadership and organizational change for implementation (LOCI): A randomized mixed method pilot study of a leadership and organization development intervention for evidence-based practice implementation. *Implementation Science* **10**, 11.

Berecki-Gisolf, J., Clay, F. J., Collie, A., and Mcclure, R. J. (2012) The impact of aging on work disability and return to work: Insights from workers' compensation claim records. *Journal of Occupational and Environmental Medicine*, **54**, 318–22.

Black, C. (2008). Working for a healthier tomorrow: Work and health in Britain. Identifies challenges and sets out recommendations for reform on health, work and wellbeing. London: The Stationary Office.

Boardman, J., and Lyon, A. (2006) Defining best practice in corporate occupational health and safety governance: HSE research report 506. London: HSE.

Böckerman, P., and Laukkanen, E. (2010) Predictors of sickness absence and presenteeism: Does the pattern differ by a respondent's health? *Journal of Occupational and Environmental Medicine*, **52**, 332–5.

Boot, C. R., Van Den Heuvel, S. G., Bültmann, U., De Boer, A. G., Koppes, L. L., and Van Der Beek, A. J. (2013) Work adjustments in a representative sample of employees with a chronic disease in the Netherlands. *Journal of Occupational Rehabilitation*, **23**, 200–8.

Christian, J., Wickizer, T., and Burton, K. (2016) A community-focused health and work service (HWS). In *SSDI Solutions: Ideas to Strengthen Social Security Disability Insurance Program*, West Conshohocken, PA, Infinity Publishing, 83–112.

Curry, L. A., Linnander, E. L., Brewster, A. L., Ting, H., Krumholz, H. M., and Bradley, E. H. (2015) Organizational culture change in US hospitals: A mixed methods longitudinal intervention study. *Implementation Science*, **10**, 29.

Damschroder, L. J., Aaron, D. C., Keith, R. E., Kirsh, S. R., Alexander, J. A., and Lowery, J. C. (2009) Fostering implementation of health services research findings into practice: A consolidated framework for advancing implementation science. *Implementation Science*, **4**, 50.

Dodek, P, Cahill, N. E., and Heyland, D. K. (2010) The relationship between organizational culture and implementation of clinical practice guidelines: A narrative review. *Journal of Parenteral and Enteral Nutrition*, **34**, 669–74.

DOH. (2017) Improving Lives: The future of work, health and disability. Presented to Parliament, Nov 2017.

Ehrhart, M., Schneider, B., and Macey, W. H. (2014) *Organizational Climate and Culture: An Introduction to Theory, Research, and Practice.* New York: Routledge.

Eisenbeiss, S. A., Van Knippenberg, D., and Boerner S.(2008) Transformational leadership and team innovation: Integrating team climate principles. *Journal of Applied Psychology,* **93**, 1438–46.

Ekberg, K., Pransky, G. S., Besen, E., Fassier, J. B, Feuerstein, M., Munir, F., et al., (2016) New business structures creating organizational opportunities and challenges for work disability prevention. *Journal of Occupational Rehabilitation*, **26**, 480–89.

Franche, R.-L., Baril, R., Shaw, W., Nicholas, M., and Loisel, P. (2005) Workplace-based return-to-work interventions: Optimizing the role of stakeholders in implementation and research. *Journal of Occupational Rehabilitation,* **15**, 525–42.

Fried, V., Bernstein, A., and Bush, M. (2012) *Multiple Chronic Conditions Among Adults Aged 45 and Older: Trends Over The Past 10 Years.* Washington DC. US Department of Health and Human Services.

Haafkens, J. A., Kopnina, H., Meerman, M. G. M., and van Dijk, F. J. H. (2011) Facilitating job retention for chronically ill employees: Perspectives of line managers and human resource managers. *BMC Health Services Research* **11**, 104.

Harden, A., Peersman, G., Oliver, S., Mauthner, M., and Oakley, A. (1999) A systematic review of the effectiveness of health promotion interventions in the workplace. *Occupational Medicine*, **49**, 540–8.

Hutting, N., Staal, J. B., Engels, J.A., Heerkens, Y. F., Detaille, S. I., and Nijhuis-Van Der Sanden, M. W. (2015) Effect evaluation of a self-management programme for employees with complaints of the arm, neck or shoulder: A randomised controlled trial. *Occupational and Environmental Medicine*, **72**, 852–61.

Jacobs, S. R., Weiner, B. J., and Bunger, A. C. (2014) Context matters: Measuring implementation climate among individuals and groups *Implementation Science*, **9**, 46.

Jones, R. A., Jimmieson, N. L., and Griffiths, A.(2005) The impact of organizational culture and reshaping capabilities on change implementation success: The mediating role of readiness for change. *Journal of Management Studies*, **42**, 361–86.

Kendall, N., Burton, A.K., Lunt, J., Mellor, N., and Daniels, K. (2015) The HSE Toolbox Developing an intervention toolbox for common health problems in the workplace. HSE Books.

Kristman, V., Shaw, W., Boot, C., Delclos, G., Sullivan, M., and Ehrhart, M. (2016) Researching complex and multi-level workplace factors affecting disability and prolonged sickness absence. *Journal of Occupational Rehabilitation*, **26**, 399–416.

Leijten, F. R., Van Den Heuvel, S. G., Ybema, J. F., Van Der Beek, A. J., Robroek, S. J., and Burdorf, A. (2014) The influence of chronic health problems on work ability and productivity at work: A longitudinal study among older employees. *Scandinavian Journal of Work, Environment and Health*, **40**, 473–82.

Lundmark, R., Hasson, H., von Thiele Schwarz, U., Hasson, D., and Tafvelin, S. (2017) Leading for change: Line managers' influence on the outcomes of an occupational health intervention. *Work and Stress*, **31**, 276–96.

Main, C. J., Nicholas, M. K., Shaw, W. S., Tetrick, L. E., Ehrhart, M. G., and Pransky, G. (2016) Implementation science and employer disability practices: Should implementation factors be imbedded in research designs? *Journal of Occupational Rehabilitation,* **26**, 448–64.

Main, C. J., and Shaw, W. S. (2016) Employer policies and practices to manage and prevent disability: Conclusion to the special issue. *Journal of Occupational Rehabilitation*, **26**, 490–98.

Martins, L. L. Organizational change and development 2011. In: Zedeck, S. (ed.), APA *Handbook of Industrial and Organizational Psychology*. Vol. **3**. Washington, DC: APA, 691–728.

Main, C., and Shaw, W. (2016). Conceptual, methodological and measurement challenges in addressing return to work in workers with musculoskeletal disorders. In: Schultz, I.Z., and Gatchel, R. (eds.) *Handbook of Return to Work: From Research to Practice*. New York: Springer, 423–57.

McCoy, K., Stinson, K., Scott, K., Tenney, L., and Newman, L.S. (2014) Health promotion in small business: A systematic review of factors influencing adoption and effectiveness of worksite wellness programs. *Journal of Occupational and Environmental Medicine*, **56**, 579–87.

Munir, F., Khan, H. T., Yarker, J., Haslam, C., Long, H., Bains, M., and Kalawsky, K. (2009) Self-management of health-behaviors among older and younger workers with chronic illness. *Patient Education and Counselling*, **77**, 109–15.

Nicholas, M. K., Watson, P. J., Linton, S. J., and Main, C. J. (2011). The identification and management of psycho- social risk factors (yellow flags) in patients with low back pain. *Physical Therapy*, **91**, 737–53.

Nishii, L. H. (2013) The benefits of climate for inclusion for gender-diverse groups. *Academy of Management Journal*, 1754–74.

OECD (2015) *Fit Mind, Fit Job: From Evidence to Practice in Mental Health and Work, Mental Health and Work*. Paris: OECD Publishing.

Pransky, G., Fassier, J. B., Besen, E., Blanck, P., Ekberg, K., Feuerstein, M. et al., (2016) Sustaining work participation across the life course: Addressing chronic health conditions in research of disability management practices. *Journal of Occupational Rehabilitation*, **26**, 465–79.

Rice, A., Smith, B. H., and Blyth, F.M. (2016) Pain and the global burden of disease. *Pain*, **157**, 791–6.

Rongen, A., Robroek, S. J., Van Lenthe, F.J., and Burdorf, A. (2013) Workplace health promotion: A meta-analysis of effectiveness. *American Journal of Preventive Medicine*, **44**, 406–15.

Schneider, B., Ehrhart, M. G., and Macey, W. H. (2013) Organizational climate and culture. *Annual Review of Psychology*, **64**, 361–88.

Schultz, I. Z., Chlebak, C. M., and Law, A. K. (2016) Bridging the gap: Evidence-informed early intervention practices for injured workers with nonvisible disabilities. In: Schultz, I. Z., and Gatchel, R. J. (eds) Handbook of Return to Work. Boston: Springer, 223–53.

Scott-Parker, S. (2014) Delivering business improvement by managing workplace adjustments as a core business process. London: Business Disability International.

Shakespeare, T., Watson, N., and Alghaib, O. A. (2016) Blaming the victim, all over again: Waddell and Aylward's biopsychosocial (BPS) model of disability. *Critical Social Policy*, **36**, 22–41.

Shaw, W. S., Main, C. J., Nicholas, M. K., Linton, S. L., Anema, J. R., and Pransky, G. (2016) Employer policies and practices to manage and prevent disability: Forword to the Special Issue. *Journal of Occupational Rehabilitation*, **26**, 394–98.

Shaw, W. S., Reme, S. E., Pransky, G., Woiszwillo, M.J., Steenstra, I., and Linton, S. J. (2013) The pain recovery inventory of concerns and expectations: A psychosocial screening instrument to identify intervention needs among patients at elevated risk of back disability. *Journal of Occupational and Environmental Medicine*, **55**, 88–94.

Shaw, W. S., van der Windt, D. A., Main C.J., Loisel, P., and Linton S. J. (2009) Now tell me about your work: The feasibility of early screening and intervention to address occupational factors ("Blue Flags") in back disability. *Journal of Occupational Rehabilitation*, **19**, 64–80.

Shore, L. M., Randel, A. E., Chung, B. G., Dean, M. A., Ehrhart, K. H., and Singh, G. (2010) Inclusion and diversity in work groups: A review and model for future research. J Manage. **37**, 1262–89.

Stansfeld, S., and Candy, B. (2006) Psychosocial work environment and mental health–a meta-analytic review. *Scandinavian Journal of Work, Environment and Health*, **32**, 443–62.

Steenstra, I. A., Verbeek, J. H., Heymans, M. W., and Bongers, P. M. (2005). Prognostic factors for duration of sick leave in patients sick listed with acute low back pain: A systematic review of the literature. *Journal of Occupational and Environmental Medicine*, **62**, 851–60.

Suff, R., and Miller, J. (2016) Growing the health and well-being agenda: From first steps to full potential. Policy report, CIPD.

Sullivan, M., Feuerstein, M., Gatchel, R. J., Linton, S., and Pransky, G. (2005). Integrating psychosocial and behavioral interventions to achieve optimal rehabilitation outcomes. *Journal of Occupational Rehabilitation*,**15**, 475–89.

Taylor, M., Marsh, G., Nicol, D., and Broadbent, P. (2017) Good Work: The Taylor review of modern work practices. Report commissioned by the UK Government.

Tetrick, L., Quick, J. C., and Gilmore, P. L. (2012) Research in organizational interventions to improve well-being: Perspectives on organizational change and development. In: Biron,

C., Karanika-Murray, M., and Cooper C. L. (eds) *Improving Organizational Interventions for Stress and Well-Being: Addressing Process and Context,* New York: Routledge/Taylor & Francis Group.

Tveito, T.H., Shaw, W. S., Huang, Y.-H., Nicholas, M., and **Wagner, G.** (2010) Managing pain in the workplace: A focus group study of challenges, strategies and what matters most to workers with low back pain. *Disability and Rehabilitation, 32,* 2035–45.

Varekamp, I., De Vries, G., Heutink, A., and Van Dijk, F. J. (2008) Empowering employees with chronic diseases; development of an intervention aimed at job retention and design of a randomised controlled trial. *BMC Health Services Research,* **8,** 224.

Vos, T., Flaxman, A. D., Naghavi, M., Lozano, R., Michaud, C., Ezzati, M., et al (2012) Years lived with disability (YLDs) for 1160 sequelae of 289 diseases and injuries 1990–2010: A systematic analysis for the Global Burden of Disease Study 2010. *Lancet,* **380,** 2163–96.

Waddell, G., and Burton, A.K. (2006) Is Work Good for Your Health and Well-being? London: The Stationery Office.

Weiner, B. J. (2009) A theory of organizational readiness for change. *Implementation Science,* **4,** 67.

Weiner, B., Amick, H., and Lee, S.-Y. (2008) Conceptualization and measurement of organizational readiness for change: A review of the literature in health services research and other fields. *Medical Care Research and Reviews,* **65,** 379–436.

Weiner, B. J., Lewis, M. A., and Linnan, L. A. (2009) Using organization theory to understand the determinants of effective implementation of worksite health promotion programs. *Health Education Research,* **24,** 292–305.

Werner, E. L., Lærum, E., Wormgoor, M. E., Lindh, E., and Indahl, A. (2007). Peer support in an occupational setting preventing LBP-related sick leave. *Occupational Medicine,* **57,** 590–5.

Wharton Business School. (2010). Why middle managers may be the most important people in your company. Retrieved from the Wharton Business School website: http://knowledge.wharton.upenn.edu.

Wickizer, T. M., Franklin, G, Fulton-Kehoe, D., Gluck, J., Mootz, R., Smith-Weller, T., et al. (2011) Improving quality, preventing disability and reducing costs in workers' compensation healthcare: A population-based intervention study. *Medical Care,* **49,** 1105–11.

Williams-Witt, K., Bultmann, U., Amick, B. C., 3rd, Munir, F., Tveito, T. H., and Anema, J. R. (2016) Workplace interventions to prevent disability from both the scientific and practice perspectives: A review of the scientific and grey literature. *Journal of Occupational Rehabilitation,* **26,** 417–33.

Wynne-Jones, G., Cowen, J., Jordan, J. L., Uthman, O., Main, C. J, Glozier, N., and van der Windt, D. (2014) Absence from work and return to work in people with back pain: A systematic review and meta-analysis. *Occupational and Environmental Medicine,* **71,** 448–56

Chapter 11

Pain, employment, and policy

Stephen Bevan

Introduction

The invisibility of pain can make it very difficult for those living with it to get recognition, support, and treatment. This is not just a challenge in workplace or clinical settings. Chronic and work-limiting pain in the working-age population often finds itself in a policy 'blind spot', falling between competing policy 'silos' for attention, resources, and, crucially, joined-up action. Here, we look at the policy 'landscape' within which those living and working with pain often have to vie for resources. We consider some of the policy 'levers' and incentives which might be used to improve both clinical and work outcomes for those living with pain, and some international examples of initiatives which may offer some solutions.

How important is workforce health to policy-makers?

It is still common to find that the health of the working-age population features only briefly in most national health strategies. This is despite compelling evidence from epidemiological and public health data that work status can be an important 'social determinant' of health and a factor in explaining several aspects of health inequality, income inequality, and social exclusion (Marmot, 2006; Black, 2008). Why then might workforce health still struggle to get the policy 'airtime' it arguably deserves?

To start with, we can consider high-level messages which health policy-makers get about where they should direct their resources. The United Nations (UN) and the World Health Organization (WHO) have quite correctly encouraged individual nations to focus on high-priority non-communicable diseases (NCDs) such as cardiovascular disease, cancer, and chronic respiratory diseases which together account for over 41 million deaths or 73.4% of all deaths annually. The 2030 'Agenda for Sustainable Development' (UN, 2018) aims to reduce by one-third preventable mortality from NCDs through prevention and treatment, with an understandable focus on supporting public health, health education, and prevention programmes in developing countries. The cost of these NCDs to health-care systems across the world is substantial, and partly explains why, with ageing populations, they are given such significant policy and resource priority.

However, one of the perverse consequences of NCDs' dominance for policy-makers, is that the conditions which cause death (mortality) tend to receive more attention that those which cause disability (morbidity). Yet the latest Global Burden of Disease data published by WHO shows, once again, that low back pain, headache disorders, depressive disorders, and diabetes occupy the top four places. The irony is that, while the top Global Burden of Disease conditions are also NCDs, they never appear on the list of Sustainable Development Goals priorities (Institute for Health Metrics and Evaluation, 2018). However, if the focus of policy-makers was more oriented to quality of life, social inclusion, health equity and building, and sustaining productive capacity of the working-age population, then the picture might be different.

Mortality is still not the main health policy concern when looking at chronic illness among working-age people. Morbidity has a far bigger impact on labour market outcomes because chronic conditions increase work absence, so-called presenteeism and work productivity loss, and cause millions of workers to leave the labour market prematurely.

Chronic conditions are associated with higher rates of sickness absence. OECD analysis of EU data shows that among 50–59-year-old workers, the number of sick days taken in a year increases steadily in most countries as the number of chronic illnesses multiply. For example, in France, the median number of days sick with no chronic disease reported was 5, with 1 chronic disease was 7 and with 2 or more was 23 (OECD 2016). This can obviously have an effect at the level of the economy but also for individual employers and businesses who are understandably keen to maximize their workforce's productive capacity. There is impact here too for individuals—in the USA men with chronic conditions work 6% fewer hours and earn 6% less than men without chronic conditions. Among women with chronic conditions, a similar working time reduction decreases earnings by 9% (OECD, 2016).

The financial consequences of this morbidity among working people is considerable. In the US labour market musculoskeletal disorders (MSDs) account for 29% of all days lost to illness and account for over $575 billion in lost productivity (2.9% of GDP). For every 100 employees, MSDs cost US employers $103k annually (Summers et al., 2015). In the EU, 44 million workers have MSDs attributable to their work at an annual cost of €240 billion each year (Bevan, 2015a; Bevan et al., 2009), a number likely to be larger when co-morbidities are taken into account.

Finally, chronic illness also leads to premature exit from the labour market either through unemployment or early retirement. Analysis of EU workers' data shows that 16% of men (and 13% of women) with chronic conditions leave work early because of chronic illness (OECD, 2016). These patterns are common across many developed economies. For example, analysis from Australia by Schofield et al. (2008) shows that, among workers over 45 years old, conditions involving pain (e.g. back pain, other MSDs, and cancer) can increase the chances of leaving the labour market prematurely by between 3.5 and 6 times, compared with other workers in the same age cohort. What emerges is, to some extent, a 'perfect storm' involving several substantial forces:

- An ageing workforce
- Longer working lives and later retirement resulting from problems with pension funding
- A growing burden of chronic ill-health in the working-age population
- Widening health inequalities.

Together, these forces affect the ability of national economies, health-care systems, and businesses to harness the productive capacity of the workforce and to maintain a high quality of life and maximize independent living among those with impaired functional and cognitive capacity. We will now look in more detail at the implications for employers and policy-makers, and the impact that both can make to mitigate the risks of ill-health in the workforce and to make improvements in health and well-being (Pfizer, 2010).

Workforce health, pain, and policy 'silos'

First, we must pause to consider how heterogeneous the group we call 'working-age people living with chronic pain' is. This is important because policy can sometimes struggle to deliver effectively for diverse groups whose needs are both highly individual and fluctuate frequently (Vaughan-Jones and Barham, 2010).

People in paid employment are often the biggest group and it is easy to see these people as sharing broadly similar characteristics compared, for example, with the unemployed. However, it does not take much interrogation of labour force statistics to identify that people in employment are very diverse. In the context of workforce health, people in permanent and full-time employment can often have the most difficulty. If we bear in mind that, among those living with some chronic musculoskeletal conditions, up to two-thirds can be the primary income earners in their household, the pressure to maintain a steady salary can be intense. This is clearly more likely to be problematic for those in low pay and low skill sectors. Many workers living with chronic pain seek to reduce their hours in order to make self-management of their condition more possible (Summers et al., 2014). While this reduction may only be temporary, it can place demands on the employer regarding productivity, reorganizing work, and maintaining service to customers, etc. From the employee's perspective, it may damage prospects of advancement if they have cause to fear that they might be regarded as unreliable by manager or co-workers. Policy-makers have to decide whether this scenario is one where regulation and employment rights might need to set a baseline of responsibilities to which employers should conform, or whether employers should have more latitude to respond or not to employees' health needs.

Within this large group of employed people, there are other groups whose needs, if they are living with chronic pain, may need to be recognized and accommodated by regulation, especially if there is a risk of discrimination. For example, those working part-time, those with caring responsibilities, and older workers, may all have varying needs to be considered and accommodated if they are to be supported in remaining in work while living with pain.

The so-called contingent workforce is another group policy-makers must consider. These people have more fluid employment patterns and contractual status, and their legal rights may also be significantly different from their employed counterparts. This is a very heterogeneous group which is becoming even more diverse as the 'gig' economy grows. A freelance IT expert with scarce skills in high demand could hardly be described as being in 'precarious' work compared with a low-paid care worker employed on very casual terms by a private sector provider, with no guaranteed hours and with a disproportionate share of 'risk' in the employment relationship. In both cases, the flexibility offered by 'contingent' work may be a good solution to the challenges of living and working with chronic pain. But, as we can see, there can be significant asymmetries of power, access, and information and control in different parts of this workforce and, once again, policy-makers have to create responses which balance the need to protect workers without placing an intolerable administrative burden on employers which, perversely, disincentivizes employing people with health problems.

The self-employed is another group whose health needs can easily be ignored. In the UK, self-employment as a proportion of total employment has grown to over 15% in recent years. However, rather than this representing the unleashing of 'animal spirits' of entrepreneurialism, a growing proportion of this group are older workers with chronic health conditions who struggle to find or keep more permanent employment. While policy-makers have generally been keen to incentivize people to set up their own businesses, they have been less ready to support those living with health conditions. The UK's Fit for Work Service, for example, which offered free telephone triage, occupational health advice, and case-managed return-to-work support for employees with 4 weeks of sickness absence, explicitly excluded the self-employed. Although this service has now been largely discontinued in England and Wales, it indicates that ill-health among the self-employed is considered by policy-makers as too complex to weave into mainstream policy initiatives. This is despite recent evidence that more than 80,000 self-employed people in the UK are moving from self-employment onto Employment Support Allowance (ESA) each year (Black and Frost, 2011).

There are other characteristics and needs of the workforce, especially that proportion living and working with chronic pain, which policy-makers must consider in formulating, executing, and evaluating policy. For example:

1. Is the pain a result of working conditions, accidents, or incidents at work, or does it arise from existing pathologies or health conditions? Although the requirement to provide support and workplace accommodations does not usually differentiate, in some countries the level and type of vocational rehabilitation intervention, even financial support, can be influenced by policy choices. For example, worker compensation schemes in parts of Europe and in Australasia, frequently provide this kind of support only to workers whose ill-health, impairment, or pain can be directly attributable to work. Those with the same degree of pain and work disability from, for example, an inflammatory condition, may not be eligible for similar compensation and support. This policy choice is governed by financial considerations and by the principle underpinning the employer's 'duty of care';

2. Is the worker living with comorbid health conditions? Although clinicians are very familiar with the concepts of multimorbidity and comorbidity, employers and policy-makers have been late to develop an understanding of what they mean for job retention and vocational rehabilitation interventions. For example, the UK Labour Force Survey only allows respondents to cite one health condition in its questions about recent sickness absence. Most employers, if they monitor sickness absence causes, only have space for one illness or impairment on what are otherwise quite sophisticated human resources systems. So, data on workforce ill-health which policy-makers and employers analyse and base financial and

other resource-allocation decisions on, over-simplifies what are really complex, comorbid, and fluctuating health challenges faced daily by thousands of working-age people living with chronic pain;

3. Is the cost of a health-care intervention which keeps someone in work worthwhile and justifiable? With advances in medical science and technology, it is now possible to intervene to sustain or even improve individuals' physical and cognitive functioning so that they can continue to work productively. But policy-makers' resource-constrained health-care systems need a reliable, transparent method of making decisions about the likely cost-effectiveness of these interventions, often requiring both ethical and health-economic considerations to be accounted for;

4. Are we clear what we mean by 'work' and which modes of working are most appropriate and beneficial for people living with chronic pain? Being 'employed' is only one model in this context: the debate about what kind of work is best remains vociferous. For example, among people with severe mental illness, there is strong evidence that competitive employment has the best therapeutic benefits. Being in a 'real' job if you have schizophrenia means that you are five times more likely to be in functional remission and have much-reduced use of health-care resources (Haro et al., 2011). This is contested by some in the 'supported employment' field who argue that volunteering, unpaid work, or even sheltered employment are the best options as these offer graduated and supported return-to-work pathways. Western policy-makers have struggled with this conundrum for decades and different countries adopt different approaches. In the UK, sheltered workshops for those with disabilities and chronic illness were closed several years ago and the competitive employment route is preferred. However, in many continental European countries sheltered employment is still widely used, as are 'quota' for employers which penalize them financially if between 3 and 6% of their workforce is not drawn from the disabled or chronically ill.

In contrast with their health policy counterparts, labour market and welfare system policy-makers in most countries want to maximize labour market participation for people with long-term, chronic illness, including chronic pain. Most have an array of 'active labour market' policies informed by a 'work first' philosophy which focuses on reducing the percentage of the population on social security or welfare benefits and maximizing those who are deriving the economic and health benefits of work, contributing not consuming tax revenues. Although there is recognition that workers with long-term illnesses and chronic pain are too often at the margins of employment, very few countries have managed to deliver comprehensive, 'joined up', and coordinated policy to tackle this.

Overview of the policy 'landscape'

There are three main areas of policy—common to most countries—which impact practically on working-age people living with chronic pain who want or need to remain active in the labour market: employment, welfare and active labour market, and health policy. In addition, and often controlling financial boundaries, is economic policy, most frequently set by finance or treasury policy-makers. These are set out in Figure 11.1.

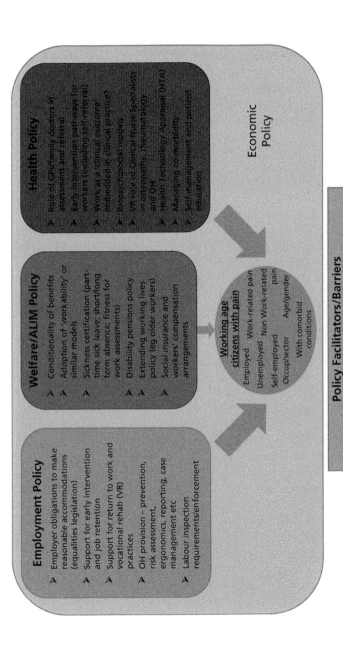

Employment Policy

➤ Employer obligations to make reasonable accommodations (equalities legislation)
➤ Support for early intervention and job retention
➤ Support for return to work and vocational rehab (VR) practices
➤ OH provision – prevention, risk assessment, ergonomics, reporting, case management etc
➤ Labour inspection requirements/enforcement

Welfare/ALIM Policy

➤ Conditionality of benefits
➤ Adoption of 'workability' or similar models
➤ Sickness certification (part-time sick leave; short/long term absence; fitness for work assessments)
➤ Disability pensions policy
➤ Extending working lives policy (eg older workers)
➤ Social insurance and workers' compensation arrangements

Health Policy

➤ Role of GP/family doctors in assessment and referral
➤ Early intervention pathways for workers (including self-referral)
➤ Work as a 'clinical outcome' embedded in clinical practice?
➤ Biopsychosocial models
➤ VR role of Clinical Nurse Specialists in osteopathy, rheumatology and OH
➤ Health Technology Appraisal (HTA)
➤ Managing co-morbidity
➤ Self-management and patient education

Working age citizens with pain

Employed   Work-related pain
Unemployed   Non Work-related pain
Self-employed   Age/gender
Occup/sector
With comorbid conditions

Economic Policy

Policy Facilitators/Barriers

Information and data sharing between agencies
Data quality and consistency
'Pooled' budgets
Medical confidentiality/disclosure practices
Working age health as a public health priority
Communication between clinicians, employers and workers
Social dialogue and partnership

Figure 11.1 Working with chronic pain—the policy 'landscape'

We look at each of these policy domains, and the facilitators and barriers to their effectiveness. First a reminder that, whatever the policy 'levers' which might be pulled at national or regional level, it is often economic policy which frames the more specific policy choices open to decision-makers. Since the 2008 global financial crisis, many national governments have been wrestling with two apparently conflicting pressures. The first is the desire to control public expenditure and to promote 'austerity' to reduce debt and borrowing. In most cases countries adopting such policies seek to reduce welfare spending, tightening the conditions giving people access to welfare and disability payments. The premise here is that greater conditionality will 'incentivize' people who are unemployed to find jobs, start paying income taxes, and reduce welfare 'dependency'. The second pressure is to control this growth in welfare payments at a time when the workforce is ageing, living longer, retiring later, and having more complex health-care needs. In some cases, this is framed as a mainly financial problem, which can make health policy-makers resistant to the pressure to divert resources to support workforce health if the main beneficiaries are social welfare budgets, employers, and individual workers. This is an especially difficult situation to support if scarce health-care resources are being allocated to other policy areas with no guarantee of a 'return' for several years.

In the next section, we will consider the many challenges facing policy-makers across the main policy areas and the choices they have to make in formulating the most appropriate policy 'mix' to support the best labour market outcomes for working-age citizens living with long-term health problems and chronic pain.

Employment policy

There are several areas where employment policy choices can improve labour market and employment outcomes for people living with chronic pain.

Most European countries and beyond place obligations on employers to make **workplace accommodations** for employees with a range of impairments and chronic conditions. Some focus on people living with disabilities in order to increase accessibility and reduce discrimination. Others have a wider scope and include people with long-term health conditions. Accommodations can include changes to the physical layout of workplaces, use of assistive technologies, adaptations to working time, and transport support. Three common concerns exist with the way some countries and their employers adopt these practices. First it is common to use the term 'reasonable' accommodations. This has unfortunate overtones: it might imply that the worker with an impairment or health condition is being allowed 'concessionary' measures which the employer judges either reasonable or unreasonable and that the worker should be grateful for whatever they are given. Second, few countries are especially sophisticated in the way they legislate or educate employers about the needs of people with hidden and fluctuating conditions, such as pain (Steadman et al., 2015). Chronic pain is a particular difficulty as it is so widespread and relies to a large extent on workers reporting it and its effects on their functional and cognitive capacity. It is also challenging as, without self-confident input from workers, many employers find it hard to know how to accommodate their work needs. Third, most countries are poor at enforcing legal provisions if employers fail to comply, either through proactive **labour inspection** or by offering protections or legal redress.

For many working-age people with chronic pain, support for **early intervention** can make a big difference to whether they can access timely support to help them remain in, or return to, work (Bevan, 2015b). Although responsive occupational health services are available to many employees in larger organizations, the majority work in smaller businesses without such support. In the UK a new service has been running, offering free telephone-based triage and return-to-work advice for workers who had been absent from work for 4 weeks or more. The 'fit for work' service was intended to intervene early enough to prevent people from falling out of work and onto welfare benefits and to provide practical **vocational rehabilitation** advice to employers. Sadly, and although referrals to the service were belatedly allowed by employers, the low numbers of workers being referred by GPs meant that the service was discontinued in 2017. Nonetheless, the service evaluation (Gloster et al., 2018), focusing on musculoskeletal conditions and common mental health conditions, did find that many of those referred benefited from receiving timely support. The loss of this service leaves a gap in UK provision but countries such as the Netherlands and parts of Scandinavia also have state-run schemes to 'encourage' employers to share responsibility for early intervention and proactive rehabilitation efforts.

An even earlier approach with strong support from emerging research but not yet embraced widely by policy-makers is the screening of **work instability** (Revicki et al., 2015). The principle is that many people with early functional impairment resulting from chronic musculoskeletal pain, for example, can be assessed to see which aspects of their job demands elevate their risk of work absence or even leaving work altogether. There are now some well-tested, validated screening tools for conditions including rheumatoid and osteoarthritis, multiple sclerosis, and some spinal injuries, which demonstrate success, contain measures of self-reported pain and benefit both employees and employers (Tang et al., 2011). Other work instability tools looking at mental health are now being developed in Sweden and—with government funding—in the UK. It is hoped that a new generation of state-sponsored early intervention tools can be developed which support early workplace interventions for workers with pain and pain-related conditions and made widely available to prevent unwanted job loss.

Another related area where some governments have chosen to impose regulation to require proactive behaviour among employers is in the field of **occupational health (OH) provision**. In Japan, for example, all employers must get an OH professional to carry out an annual risk assessment of the workplace and key workers (Zheltoukhova et al., 2012). While the requirements are less onerous for smaller employers, it remains a national provision which, although focusing more on physical than mental health, does direct employers towards their workers' health and productive capacity. In the Netherlands, the government has fashioned perhaps more 'interventionist' sickness and rehabilitation law. Under its provisions—where 'reintegration' is the dominant policy objective—employers must pay up to at least 70% of the worker's pay for up to 104 weeks of sickness or disability. In practice, most employers pay 100% of the salary for year 1 and 70% in year 2. In addition to the sick pay rule, employers must use an OH professional to deliver a 'return-to-work' plan for the worker. These policies mean that employers and the government have a common interest in developing good working conditions and encouraging employers to invest effort and resources into prevention, risk assessment, ergonomics, reporting, case management, and re-habilitation across a range of health conditions.

Of course, **enforcement** of employer's legal obligations has to be part of the policy 'mix' available to governments. In Europe, enforcement is 'patchy': Scandinavian countries have a better record than most of making sure businesses comply with their legal duty of care. Enforcement capacity now needs to move beyond traditional areas such as health and safety. In the UK, with the publication of new regulations on so-called Good work standards (Taylor, 2017), there is now recognition that good quality jobs are beneficial to health (Henseke, 2018). To support enforcing these standards a new Director of Labour Market Enforcement (Metcalf, 2018) has been appointed, signalling that employers must take their legal and moral duty to promote workforce well-being seriously.

Welfare and active labour market policy

Policy-makers globally have to balance providing a health and welfare 'safety net' and support infrastructure for working-age people with chronic ill-health, and the expectation that these citizens will remain economically active where possible. This balancing act centres on several tensions. First, is a crude and sometimes simplistic conundrum—that people at work tend to contribute more to national revenue (through taxation) and productive capacity than those who are not working (who are net resource consumers). Second is a more clinical challenge—how to assess ro-bustly and equitably whether functional or cognitive limitations prevent a person from working at all or, if they can work, how to match them to suitable, fulfilling work. This is especially important for those living with hidden and fluctuating impairments, such as chronic pain. Third is how to target interventions which support job retention and return-to-work which optimize support and minimize compulsion.

These tensions are easy to politicize and no developed economy has managed to escape controversy over the way that those at the margins of the labour market as a result of their health should be treated. As a result, issues such as the '**condition-ality**' of benefits, the calibration and targeting of '**active labour market policy**', and the best ways to 'incentivize' people with health challenges to engage fully with work, have become as much to do with political ideology as with science. Indeed, this is an area where the debate about 'evidence-based policy' has raged for several decades (Strassheim and Kettunen, 2014).

One problem is that, in setting national policy in this field, the importance of indi-vidual differences and fluctuations in health or symptoms can easily be underplayed or ignored. This can lead some policy measures to imply that being 'fit' for work is amenable to a simple binary judgement which can govern access to support, wel-fare payments, and care. Some countries, however, try to resolve this problem with more personalized and flexible approaches; the Scandinavian '**workability**' model (Ilmarinen, 2009) is a good example. As the workforce ages and experiences more chronic illness, approaches which help redesign work around the capabilities and strengths of individuals will help vocational rehabilitation, job retention, productivity, and engagement. Additionally, policies governing sickness certification can have the unwanted effect of making primary care physicians the arbiter of a patient's fitness to work, a role which many resent and argue they are not trained to perform. Although it has not been entirely successful, the UK '**Fit Note**' has, since 2010, been an attempt to make the conversation about fitness to work and workplace adjustments a three-way exchange between doctor, patient/worker, and employer, focusing less on what workers cannot do and more on what tasks they can still perform if appropriate support in the workplace was available (Dorrington et al., 2018).

Another increasingly relevant aspect of welfare policy is the need to consider measures which encourage more older workers to stay at work beyond normal retirement age. This is driven partly by demographic pressures and by the need to reduce state pension costs by **extending working lives** even among older workers living with chronic illness and pain. This imperative has led to more research and policy activity to support older workers and employers to work together to make modern workplaces more accommodating towards those with long-term conditions (Palmer et al., 2017).

Health policy

The role of health-care policy and of health-care professionals is gaining increased prominence among policy-makers seeking to 'join up' initiatives which prioritize employment opportunities for working-age citizens with long-term and chronic health challenges. A key principle, now being more widely embraced, is that **work should be regarded as a clinical outcome**—especially if staying in or returning to work is an important priority for the patient and if work might have positive therapeutic or rehabilitative benefits for them.

Using only clinical criteria there is a clear case for **early intervention** in most cases of chronic pain. Among workers living with pain there is the added benefit of improving both pain management and work outcomes. For example, early referral of an employee to appropriate medical or occupational health support may make the biggest difference to that employee's chances of remaining in or returning successfully to work. Indeed, studies show (Bevan, 2015b) that early intervention for people with MSDs can:

♦ Reduce sick leave and lost work productivity by more than 50%. Early intervention is commonly more cost effective than 'usual care' (Goetzel and Ozminkowski, 2008);

♦ Reduce health-care costs by up to two-thirds (Theodore et al., 2015);

♦ Reduce disability benefits costs by up to 80% (Abasolo et al., 2005);

♦ Reduce the risk of permanent work disability and job loss by up to 50% (Abasolo et al., 2005);

♦ Reduce the risk of developing a co-morbid mental illness (McGee and Ashby, 2010);

♦ Deliver societal benefits by supporting people with work-limiting chronic conditions to optimize their functional capacity and remain active at work and maintain economic independence (Vermeulen et al., 2013).

Prioritizing early intervention also means being able to deliver at least some elements of vocational rehabilitation, which can also involve risk assessment and prevention. This means that a solid, joined-up approach to workplace health which has early intervention, job redesign, and vocational rehabilitation at its core may be better than any single intervention, no matter how eye-catching or well-branded. It is increasingly common, though some still argue too slow, for patients to have access to self-referral services to physiotherapy, for example. In the UK 30% of GP consultations are for musculoskeletal pain and earlier referral to a physiotherapist can improve access and work outcomes and can free up GP resources—costing up to 25% less than a GP referral (Holdsworth et al., 2007).

Another aspect of health policy which is rarely considered in the context of employment is **Health Technology Appraisal** (HTA). This is the process by which 'cost effectiveness' of new drug therapies or medical devices are assessed, usually by calculating how many additional Quality Adjusted Life Years (QALYs) for patients they might deliver. The QALY is a standardized measure used by health economists to measure the economic value of improvements in clinical or quality of life outcomes which a medical intervention might bring about. For example, biologic therapies have transformed the lives of some people living with autoimmune conditions such as inflammatory bowel disease (e.g. ulcerative colitis and Crohn's disease), rheumatoid arthritis, and ankylosing spondylitis. Each of these conditions can involve fluctuating flares of inflammation, fatigue and chronic pain, yet biologic/biosimilar drug therapies can arrest the progression of these conditions, can restore function, and allow the resumption of 'activities of daily living'—including employment. Access to—and reimbursement for—these often-expensive treatments is governed by HTA, and the various national agencies which conduct these appraisals have sometimes different approaches to the inclusion of 'work' or 'productivity' dimensions (Barham and Bevan, 2012).

In the UK, the National Institute for Health and Care Excellence (NICE) conducts a traditional cost-per QALY analysis. In general, if a new intervention costs less than £40k for each additional QALY, it is likely to be approved for reimbursement and wider use in the NHS and simultaneously judged as likely to deliver value for money to taxpayers. Policy-makers around the world set the terms of reference and the cost per QALY thresholds used by HTA agencies, and some specify that if a medical intervention can help a patient stay in or return to work (and pay tax, not use welfare payments, and add to the productive capacity of the economy), then that economic benefit can be included in HTA assessment. Other agencies are discouraged or prohibited from including these factors in HTA for fear that doing so implies that health-care resource allocation should favour those of working-age over children or the elderly. In the UK, the Department of Health and Social Care has been reluctant to allow NICE to routinely include work or productivity assumptions in its economic evaluations, whereas the Netherlands routinely does (Krol, 2012). One argument here is that, if countries wish to improve labour market participation among people living with chronic pain, it would be self-defeating not to allow HTA to include work participation and productivity benefits when deciding who gets access to medical interventions which improve work ability.

Policy facilitators and barriers

A familiar challenge in the health and work policy arena is that of **siloed thinking and siloed budgeting**. It is argued that real improvements in workforce health are unlikely to happen unless we find ways of getting stakeholders with overlapping interests to collaborate more (McDaid, 2012). Officials in finance ministries around the world are frequently told by advocates of 'spend to save' interventions that if they let the health system spend (invest) more in workforce health interventions (e.g. early interventions, rehabilitation, etc.) then the savings to the labour/social welfare ministry in reduced welfare payments would deliver an attractive 'return on investment (ROI)'. However, there at least three pragmatic difficulties here:

1. Finance ministers invariably needs a higher quality of 'proof' that the promised ROI will materialize than is often available. They might concede that there are latent benefits but they will hardly ever accept that these benefits can be 'cashed-out' in the way their advocates claim. They are probably right to take this position.

2. Ministerial budgets are rarely diverted to projects whose benefits will accrue mainly to ministers in other departments—especially in time of austerity. It is not that ministers are ideologically opposed to collaboration in principle. It is just that there are no incentives (but plenty of criticism) if they allocate funding to such ostensibly risky ventures.

3. Even if the ROI from a 'pooled' collaboration is highly likely to be delivered, and even if Ministers in different Departments do forge an energetic, committed collaboration, if the results of initiatives cannot be guaranteed to deliver within an electoral cycle, then it will be harder to get them off the ground.

In reality—and compared with the challenge of getting a number of ministries to join forces and budgets—collaboration between local stakeholders (including employers) and agencies of government may be a more realistic model worth exploring in more detail, especially as a few models and templates in the workforce health domain exist already. Box 11.1 shows a Swedish example illustrating that, with enabling legislation, budget-pooling at local level can deliver better employment outcomes for people with long-term health conditions.

So how could this approach be adapted for other countries and how could employers be involved more directly as partners or stakeholders? We could pilot a number of budget-pooling models involving matched funding between local agencies (including private sector providers where they can add value) and employers—perhaps managed through public health agencies, local authorities (municipalities), and employer or trade bodies and unions. These pilots would target evidence-based interventions in workplaces and among those claiming disability benefits with both a public health and workplace health focus. They would test the mechanisms for budget-pooling, and the outcomes of specific local job retention and rehabilitation pilots on work outcomes. The Welsh Government has started to develop approaches to joint working across agencies which offer opportunities to improve employment outcomes for workers with health problems (Bevan, 2018).

Even if employment, welfare, and health policy are aligned sufficiently to prioritize the needs of working-age people with chronic and painful conditions, a key barrier can be employers' willingness to play a full part in providing good quality work, accommodating workplaces, and the leadership required to deliver sustainable employment

Box 11.1 Local budget-pooling for vocational rehabilitation in Sweden

In Sweden, cross-sectoral initiatives have been the subject of much evaluation. The SOCSAM scheme allowed social insurance and social services to voluntarily move up to 5% of their budgets, along with a matched contribution from health services, to a pooled budget to jointly manage rehabilitation services to help individuals on long-term sick leave return to employment. It was evaluated in eight localities and compared with experience elsewhere in the country where schemes were not introduced. Along with funding, joint financial management arrangements were set up, helping to foster the development of joint services and a more holistic approach to activities. The evaluation found that interdisciplinary collaboration between health and social care professionals improved compared to control areas (Hultberg, Lonnroth, and Allebeck, 2003). This Swedish experience also suggests joint funding arrangements and collaboration at local or regional level, where institutional structures are closer to stakeholders and have a better understanding of local problems, can be effective. Following evaluation, a new scheme to support cooperation across these sectors was rolled out on a voluntary basis nationwide (Stahl et al., 2010).

Since the early 1990s, there have been extensive experiments in Sweden with inter-sectoral collaboration in the field of vocational rehabilitation. As in many other countries, the responsibility for rehabilitation is divided between welfare institutions belonging to different sectors and levels of society. Between 1993 and 1997, there was an experiment where resources for rehabilitation were transferred from the national social insurance system to the health-care system in five localities, with the aim of reducing the costs of sickness benefits. Between 1994 and 2002 the experiment was extended in eight municipalities to include social services and the national employment service. In this experiment, there was financial coordination between the different institutions involved and inter-sectoral collaboration in cross-boundary groups or teams. Both of these experiments were evaluated and initial positive results led to the 2003 Act on Financial Coordination of Rehabilitation Measures. Although not binding, this legislation made it possible for institutions in the rehabilitation field—the national employment service, the national social insurance administration, the regional health services, and municipal social services—to form local associations for financial coordination.

Evaluation studies of these arrangements show that significant reductions in long-term sick leave can be achieved by local collaboration and financial coordination. While more evidence needs to be gathered, the improvement in job retention and return to work—especially for people with MSDs—is encouraging.

and progression opportunities. So how might policy incentivize employers to do more in this domain?

There is a large literature on the business benefits to employers of investing more in workforce health (Cooper and Bevan, 2014). Despite this, about a quarter of employers (Buck Consultants, 2014) still argue that, beyond their basic legal duty of care, workforce health is not their concern. So how can policy-makers incentivize more employers to go beyond this legal minimum? How can businesses be encouraged to go further than the so-called fruit and Pilates approach to workplace health promotion (Bevan and Bajorek, 2018) to adopt more sustainable and evidence-based approaches which can accommodate the needs of workers with chronic, fluctuating, and painful conditions? Following is a brief discussion of measures which policy-makers around the world have considered when attempting to encourage or incentivize employers to do more to promote workforce health and well-being.

Fiscal incentives

A barrier to the implementation of workplace health and well-being programmes is the limited funding which employers can make available for this. Many have questioned whether some aspects of the tax system discourage employers from investing in early interventions, even if they do recognize advantages. The argument for providing tax incentives for health and well-being programmes suggests that if such initiatives become tax free, then the demand for them will rise. From an employer's perspective, if they feel that the government wants them to implement initiatives that go beyond 'benefits in kind' or their legal duty of care, and, to have a wider societal impact and public health benefits, then perhaps the bargain should involve some help or a 'nudge' from the government itself. This may encourage organizations who might not have considered health and well-being interventions to do so.

The issue of tax incentives in the UK was also raised in the Sickness Absence Review (Black and Frost, 2011), so is not a new idea. Policy-makers have in the past questioned whether tax incentives would be cost-effective in relation to workplace health and well-being interventions mainly due to the 'deadweight' argument: i.e. employers who are already investing in workplace interventions for health will continue to do so regardless of the incentive and would effectively be receiving a subsidy for what they are already doing. For tax breaks to be considered seriously, we need to demonstrate their effectiveness, for example through evidence from other countries that have shown that they do have a positive impact on workplace health and well-being, or through longitudinal research testing the relationship between tax incentives, organizational investments in health and well-being programmes (plus the sustainability of these programmes over time), and employee outcomes. There is also a need for further evidence of the use of tax breaks on the 'net' increase in employers adopting evidence-based interventions and not just as a subsidy for existing initiatives.

Responsible procurement

If governments wish to highlight the importance of workplace health and well-being, then there is an argument that public sector organizations should apply the 'most economically advantageous tender' principle when undertaking public procurement, and ensure that they procure from organizations with reputable organizational health, safety, and well-being policies. Public sector clients could query a supplier's health and safety record, their level of sickness absence, their incidence of mental illness and physical illness, what level of investment in workplace health and well-being has been undertaken, and what other interventions have been implemented. Policy-makers may be resistant to this approach on cost grounds, especially if this reduces competitive intensity and results in rising public sector costs. However, if labour standards improve for organizations that are encouraged to implement health and well-being schemes, then costs elsewhere (e.g. health costs and health risks) may reduce.

Regulation

A more interventionist approach to encouraging employers to provide health and well-being interventions is to regulate which measures they must provide. This approach would provide more weight than current guidelines, such as those from NICE guidance and the Health and Safety Executive management standards in the UK, by making the provision of certain interventions compulsory or by requiring employers to report on their use. The main problem here is compliance. In Japan, 51.9% of enterprises with 1–4 employees, about 42% of enterprises with 5–9 employees, and 20% of organizations with 10–49 employees did not conduct the special health examinations required (Furuki et al., 2006). In particular, as highlighted in the Sickness Absence Review, this approach generally works best in countries with more statist welfare systems, whereas the UK has a more libertarian model (Black and Frost, 2011). It would therefore require a significant cultural shift, with employers starting to associate the health and wellbeing of employees with ROI, in order to achieve significant compliance.

Reporting requirements

If government understands and accepts that employment quality and employee health and well-being have implications for business performance and social outcomes, then there may be a case for increased regulation in what organizations should disclose and report regarding health and well-being practices they undertake (Business in the Community, 2013). Developing a regulatory regime where reporting is required will subject organizational practices to greater public scrutiny and may encourage behaviours which make employer activities more robust.

Making pain and employment and policy 'fit for purpose'

A complex policy architecture must be constructed and sustained to maximize labour market participation among working-age people with chronic ill-health. This means:

1. Defining what good work outcomes mean for people with fluctuating, invisible, and painful health conditions;
2. Aligning several, often conflicting, aspects of employment, welfare, health, and economic policy to support people with health conditions to participate fully in the evolving world of work;

3. Overcoming a range of challenging barriers such as stigma, low expectations, siloed budgeting (and thinking), and occasional recalcitrance among employers to promote work as a key policy and clinical care outcome.

Looking internationally, there are now several examples of thoughtful, well-constructed, and well-evaluated policy interventions which demonstrate 'what works' and when. More effort is needed to share both the research evidence which enhances our understanding of the determinants of successful design and implementation and a lively, rich exchange of experiences among practitioners to ensure that lessons from successful interventions are shared and disseminated widely. The proportion of the working-age population likely to live with chronic pain is growing. Unless we improve the way the policy landscape works for them all, their ability to participate fully in future labour markets will be severely constrained.

References

Abasolo, L., Blanco, M., Bachiller, J., Candelas, G., Collado, P., Lajas, C., et al. (2005) Health system program to reduce work disability related to musculoskeletal disorders. *Annals of Internal Medicine*, **143**, 404–14.

Barham, L., and Bevan, S. (2012) *Making Work Count—How Health Technology Assessment Can Keep Europeans in Work*. Lancaster: The Work Foundation.

Bevan, S. (2015a) Economic impact of musculoskeletal disorders (MSDs) on work in Europe, *Best Practice and Research Clinical Rheumatology*, **29**, 356–73.

Bevan, S. (2015b) *Back to Work: Exploring the Benefits of Early Interventions Which Help People with Chronic Illness Remain in Work, Fit for Work Europe*. London: The Work Foundation.

Bevan, S. (2018) *Improving Health and Employment Outcomes Through Joint Working*. Cardiff: Public Policy Institute for Wales.

Bevan, S., and Bajorek, Z. (2018) Why 'good work' trumps fruit and Pilates evangelism every time. *HR Magazine*, 29 October.

Bevan, S., Quadrello, T., McGee, R., Mahdon, M., Vavrovsky, A., and Barham, L. (2009) *Fit for Work? Musculoskeletal Disorders in the European Workforce*, London: The Work Foundation.

Black, C. (2008). *Working for a Healthier Tomorrow. Dame Carol Black's Review of the Health of Britain's Working Age Population*. London: Department for Work and Pensions.

Black, C., and Frost, D. (2011) *Health at Work—An Independent Review of Sickness Absence*. London: The Stationary Office.

Buck Consultants. (2014) Global wellness survey. Online. Available at: https://www.globalhealthyworkplace.org/tag/buck-consultants-global-wellness-survey/

Business in the Community (BITC) (2013). *BITC Public Reporting Guidelines. Employee Engagement and Wellbeing*. London: Business in the Community.

Cooper, C., and Bevan, S. (2014) Business benefits of a healthy workforce. In Day, A., Kelloway, K., and Hurrell, J. (eds), *Workplace Well-being: How to Build Psychologically Healthy Workplaces*, Chichester: Wiley, 27–49.

Dorrington, S., Roberts, E., Mykletun, A., Hatch, S., Madan, I., and Hotopf, M. (2018) Systematic review of fit note use for workers in the UK. *Occupational and Environmental Medicine*, **75**, 530–9.

Furuki, K., Hirata, M., and Kage, A. (2006) Nationwide survey of occupational health activities in small-scale enterprises in Japan. *Industrial Health,* **44**, 150–4.

Gloster, R., Marvell, R., and Huxley, C. (2018) *Fit for Work: Final Report of a Process Evaluation.* Brighton: Institute for Employment Studies.

Goetzel, R. Z., and Ozminkowski, R. J. (2008) The health and cost benefits of work site health-promotion programs. *Annual Review of Public Health,* **29**, 303–23.

Haro, J., Novick, D., Bertsch, J., Karagianis, J., Dossenbach, M., and Jones, P. (2011) Cross-national clinical and functional remission rates: Worldwide Schizophrenia Outpatient Health Outcomes (W-SOHO) study. *British Journal of Psychiatry,* **199**, 194–201.

Henseke, G. (2018) Good jobs, good pay, better health? The effects of job quality on health among older European workers. *European Journal of Health Economics,* **19**, 59–73.

Holdsworth, L., Webster, V., and McFadyen, A., (2007) What are the costs to NHS Scotland of self-referral to physiotherapy? Results of a national trial. *Physiotherapy,* **93**, 3–11.

Hultberg, E., Lonnroth, K., and Allebeck, P. (2003) Co-financing as a means to improve collaboration between primary health care, social insurance and social service in Sweden. A qualitative study of collaboration experiences among rehabilitation partners. *Health Policy,* **64**, 143–52.

Ilmarinen, J. (2009) Work ability—A comprehensive concept for occupational health research and prevention. *Scandinavian Journal of Work and Environmental Health,* **35**, 1–5.

Krol, M. (2012) *Productivity Costs in Economic Evaluations.* Rotterdam: Erasmus University.

Marmot, M. (2006) *Status Syndrome: How Your Social Standing Directly Affects Your Health and Life Expectancy.* London: Bloomsbury.

Metcalf, D. (2018) *United Kingdom Labour Market Enforcement Strategy 2018/19,* London: The Stationary Office.

McDaid, D. (2012) Joint budgeting: Can it facilitate intersectoral action? In: McQueen, D., Wismar, M., Lin, V., Jones, C. M., and Davies, M. (eds) *Intersectoral Governance for Health in All Policies: Structures, Actions and Experiences,* Copenhagen: The European Observatory on Health Systems and Policies, 111–28.

McGee, R., and Ashby, K. (2010) *Body and Soul: Exploring the Connection Between Physical and Mental Health Conditions,* London: The Work Foundation.

OECD. (2016) *Health at a Glance.* Paris: OECD.

Palmer, K.T., D'Angelo, S., Harris, E.C., Linaker, C., Sayer, A.A., Gale, C.R., et al. (2017) Sleep disturbance and the older worker: Findings from the Health and Employment after Fifty study. *Scandinavian Journal of Work and Environmental Health,* **43**, 136–45.

Pfizer. (2010) *Pain Proposal: Improving the Current and Future Management of Chronic Pain. A European Consensus Report.* London: Pfizer.

Revicki, D., Ganguli, A., Kimel, M., Roy, S., Chen, N., Safikhani, S., and Cifaldi, M. (2015) Reliability and validity of the work instability scale for rheumatoid arthritis. *Value in Health,* **18**, 1008–15.

Schofield, D., Shrestha, R., Passey, M., Earnest, A., and Fletcher, S. (2008) Chronic disease and labour force participation among older Australians. *Medical Journal of Australia,* **189**, 447–50.

Stahl, C., Svensson, T., Petersson, G., and Ekberg, K. (2010) A matter of trust? A study of coordination of Swedish stakeholders in return-to-work. *Journal of Occupational Rehabilitation* **20**, 299–310.

Steadman, K., Shreeve, V., and **Bevan, S.** (2015) *Fluctuating Conditions, Fluctuating Support: Improving Organisational Resilience to Fluctuating Conditions in the Workforce.* Lancaster: The Work Foundation.

Strassheim, H., and **Kettunen, P.** (2014) When does evidence-based policy turn into policy-based evidence? Configurations, contexts and mechanisms, *Evidence and Policy*, **10**, 259–77.

Summers, K., Bajorek, Z., and **Bevan, S.** (2014) *Self-management of Chronic Musculoskeletal Disorders and Employment.* Lancaster: The Work Foundation.

Summers, K., Jinnett, K., and **Bevan, S** (2015) *Musculoskeletal Disorders, Workforce Health and Productivity in the United States*, Lancaster: The Work Foundation.

Tang, K., Beaton, D., Boonen, A., Gignac, M., and **Bombardier, C.** (2011) Measures of work disability and productivity: Rheumatoid Arthritis Specific Work Productivity Survey (WPS-RA), Workplace Activity Limitations Scale (WALS), Work Instability Scale for Rheumatoid Arthritis (RA-WIS), Work Limitations Questionnaire (WLQ), and Work Productivity and Activity Impairment Questionnaire (WPAI). *Arthritis Care and Research*, **63**(S11), S337–49.

Taylor, M. (2017) *Good Work: The Taylor Review of Modern Working Practices.* London: Department of Business, Energy and Industrial Strategy (BEIS).

The Institute for Health Metrics and Evaluation (IHME). (2018) Global Burden of Disease. Online. Available at: http://www.healthdata.org/gbd

Theodore, B., Mayer, T., and **Gatchel, R.** (2015) Cost-effectiveness of early versus delayed functional restoration for chronic disabling occupational musculoskeletal disorders. *Journal of Occupational Rehabilitation*, **25**, 303–15.

United Nations. (2018) Sustainable Development Goals. Online. Available at: https://www.un.org/sustainabledevelopment/sustainable-development-goals/

Vaughan-Jones, H., and **Barham, L.** (2010) *Healthy Work: Evidence into Action.* BUPA.

Vermeulen, S., Heymans, M., Anema, J., Schellart, A., van Mechelen, W., and **van der Beek, A.** (2013) Economic evaluation of a participatory return-to-work intervention for temporary agency and unemployed workers sick-listed due to musculoskeletal disorders. *Scandinavian Journal of Work and Environmental Health*, **39**, 46–56.

Zheltoukhova, K., Bevan, S., and **Waterson, H.** (2012) *Fit for Work? Musculoskeletal Disorders and the Japanese Labour Market.* London: The Work Foundation.

Chapter 12

Discussion

Elaine Wainwright and Christopher Eccleston

Introduction

Pain takes a significant toll on individuals, on families, and on society as a whole. In part that damage is mediated by the loss of occupation, and the unwelcome distortion of roles, of financial capability, and of purpose. We judged that the effects of work on pain, and equally of pain on work, are becoming invisible. There is too little serious academic study on what are major drivers of modern society and well-being. We have drawn together leaders in their field to teach us how we can best think about the complexities of the relations between pain and occupation. We asked our writers to discuss how pain interacts with specific parts of the life-course and its attendant occupations, such as being a child or parent, going to school with pain or teaching a child in pain, experiencing emerging adulthood, being a worker in pain, or managing one's later life production. Our research leaders have discussed what the main issues are, and how we might improve the situation for stakeholders, but also how we might fundamentally re-imagine and re-conceptualize our response to the many current challenges in the field of pain and work.

In this last chapter, we discuss several key overarching themes. We use the contribution to theory and practice the chapters make to inform a conceptual and analytical map of the forces of change in work, occupation, and pain management. Our findings have implications for research and policy at macro and micro levels. We suggest directions for research and policy that could positively impact the lives of people in pain who are negotiating the worlds of work. We mean 'work' in the sense of employment, and as occupation in the broader sense of being busy at school, emerging into the workforce, as an older person and, in all cases, working out how to live a life with chronic or intermittent pain. Essentially, therefore, we are providing a means of reconceptualizing relations between work and pain and additionally, we are overlaying precise research directions. Here we have presented expert analyses not only of the problems, but also of how we can innovate, as we find better solutions for managing one of the most significant health burdens of our age.

A major consideration throughout has been the value of work. What is 'good' work for working-age adults when they have pain? All of the following is what we know which applies to the workplace, but most of it has not yet been considered in the context of how pain may alter one's subjective life course and engagement with work as a millennial, contingent, or older worker. There is strong agreement that rather than seeing work as something from which the patient should be protected (which still happens more than it should, as discussed by Sullivan, Pimentel, and Paré in Chapter 9) good work should be regarded as a health outcome. This principle is usually considered from the point of view of the patient, especially if returning to work sustainably is important for them, since it is likely to confer improvements in both pain management and work outcomes, as discussed by Bevan (Chapter 11). The principle is also considered important from the point of view of long-term gains for society in terms of growing a healthy, contributing population who can look after each other as the age pyramid slopes ever more steeply to those at the older end of the spectrum. Whilst this perspective of good work as a health outcome could be seen as a trope, as a way to get armies of patients, health-care professionals, and employers to work together to get people back to work sustainably, the benefits of 'good' work are so numerous and profound for the worker, that 'good' work itself can literally be viewed as a health outcome.

According to the seminal review by Waddell and Burton in 2006, work which occurs in physically and psychologically 'safe and accommodating' environments is good for our health and well-being (Waddell and Burton, 2006, p. ix) and this can include people who are living with ongoing pain. This appears to be true today, as we refine our knowledge of what 'safe and accommodating' work constitutes for people in pain. As Main and Shaw discuss in Chapter 10, there is evidence for some workplace prognostic factors when thinking about pain. For example, they highlight how we know that occupational factors in back disability include physical and psychological demands, as well as social and managerial factors. Worker perceptions of work and working conditions have been identified as potential obstacles to optimal function and to recovery (Shaw et al., 2009).

There is also evidence to suggest that if one has a manager, they are likely to be key to the quality of our experience of work, modern technology notwithstanding (as discussed by Bevan in Chapter 11). This agrees with the argument presented by Calnan and Douglass in Chapter 2 that changes in work, whilst immense, are not as fundamental as some commentators assume, and that we need to pay more attention to line management structures and resources than we do at present. Relatedly, Main and Shaw in Chapter 10 show that organizational leadership is key if we are to have successful implementation of interventions designed to sustain working lives for people in pain.

Main and Shaw (Chapter 10) discuss the conceptual model which has been proposed as part of an intervention toolbox designed to reduce work-relevant common health problems and reduce sick leave for such complaints, and this is also relevant to pain-related work limitations (Kendall et al., 2015). The model has three areas:

1. good work: essentially, the provision of good jobs including supportive workplaces for when people are ill;

2. good jobs: here, the key points are that such jobs have balanced demands, and are safe, with effective line managers and opportunities for skill development;

3. supportive workplaces: including senior management commitment, offering temporary modification, and liaison with health-care professionals.

The model integrates current theory and empirical evidence to suggest how to create healthy workplaces for people with common health problems, which is directly relevant to those living with chronic pain; it should be an important future part of testing what constitutes good workplaces for people in pain.

We think attention should be paid to Main and Shaw's own work, as described in their chapter, which leads them to suggest reconceptualizing pain-related work limitations as a problem of **sustained re-integration into work** (Chapter 10). This conceptualization means we must consider traditional work disability perspectives but combine them with contextual analyses of the nature of the workplace. Before an intervention is introduced, the instigators should conduct a re-engagement analysis, in which they would consider the characteristics of the targeted population, the type of work, and working conditions, and consider what to measure and how to measure it, using advances in implementation science. At all times, instigators should perform the difficult but necessary task of finding consensus between clinical and organizational objectives so that all relevant stakeholders really are engaged with the whole process.

Bevan (Chapter 11) also discusses evidence that early intervention is helpful in most cases of someone suffering with chronic pain, improving both pain management and work outcomes: early referral to medical or occupational health support may make the biggest difference to the chance of the worker staying in, or returning to, work. Early intervention enables some vocational rehabilitation elements to be delivered. The chapters by Bevan and Main and Shaw agree that a joined-up approach to workplace well-being, which includes awareness of job redesign needs, vocational rehabilitation, and engages all stakeholders directly, is needed.

If we now turn from a consideration of work to occupation, then the forms of occupation discussed in this book include being a child in pain, parenting a child in pain, being a parent who themselves suffers with a painful condition, whether or not one's child does, being engaged in the particular work of being a millennial, or conducting one's own later life production. Just as 'good' work can be seen as a health outcome, including for people in pain, can these forms of occupation also usefully be seen as health outcomes in their own right, if, to borrow from the literature on employment, the occupation is physiologically and psychologically safe?

For the child in pain, the main occupations are likely to be personal identity development and schooling, which are linked by the critical role school attendance plays, in academic, personal, and social development. Evidence to date (discussed in Chapter 5) strongly suggests that the child in pain who can engage with school will, unsurprisingly, do better across a range of health and academic outcomes. However, there is a small but important caveat. Caes and Logan show that how teachers and schools respond to a child in pain is critical yet has hardly been researched, and that from what we do know, schools are under-resourced in this regard. Just as the quality and appropriateness of individual line manager and organizational approaches to the worker in pain vary, so may individual teacher and school responses to the child in pain. We simply do not know enough about how schools currently support children in pain. This is remarkable in 2019, given what is known about the long-term effects of poor engagement with school for children with ongoing pain. We are learning more about how individual teachers and schools can support the child in pain, summarized as provision of official training and resources on pain management, and establishing effective communication channels between the school staff, parents, and health-care team (Logan and Curran, 2005; Tarpey et al., 2018). We need to know more about optimum responses and interactions and to map these onto current resources in different educational systems. We should also be ambitious and consider how systems and settings might change, bearing in mind real-world constraints but also seeking to improve these where possible. For example in Chapter 2, Calnan and Douglass show that for all school leavers, the increasing complexity of the labour market requires more authentic careers provision (Mann and Huddleston, 2017) and this is likely to be doubly so for the young person negotiating this complex market whilst also managing fluctuating levels of pain. So, in summary, 'safe and appropriate' schooling, as occupation, is a positive entity for the child in pain, but we under-resource future research in how to maximize such safety and appropriateness at our peril.

Parenting, whether parent, child, both, or neither has a pain condition, can be uplifting, challenging, and provoking. Parents who have a child living with pain might have to relinquish traditional parental roles and find new ones, and they might also need to change their working patterns or even give up work and hobbies. Can parents be helped with re-conceptualizing how what they are doing whilst parenting a child in pain is valuable, in the way that a worker with chronic pain might need to re-conceptualize how any new working patterns or roles they take on to accommodate their pain is valuable? Values might lie in quite different arena from before and this can be hard to accommodate as part of one's identity as parent, or worker. As Jordan and Jaaniste discuss in Chapter 4, whilst there is limited evidence for treatment effectiveness of parental-focused interventions, there are some promising results from family-based cognitive behavioural therapy and parental problem-solving therapy (PPST) within the specific context of paediatric chronic pain. For example, Jordan and Jaaniste discuss how Palermo et al. (2016) showed that PPST resulted in significantly reduced levels of parental catastrophizing and improved levels of parental physical functioning post intervention with some maintained improvements at follow up. Clearly, this is a promising direction to explore further.

For the parent who suffers with pain and also works, there is almost a double jeopardy as they have to negotiate their role as parent who may not be able to do all they desire with their child, in addition to managing some level of incapacity at work. Jordan and Jaaniste very ably discuss parents and parenting studies in Chapter 4, and many of our chapters discuss being a worker with pain, but no studies we have seen to date consider how to negotiate being a parent in pain as well as simultaneously negotiating one's role as a worker in pain. Furthermore, as Jordan and Jaaniste note, the majority of the parenting literature focuses on mothers; we know far less about fathers, and virtually nothing about step-parents, or same-sex parenting couples, grandparents, or others in a parenting role. Nothing is known about how difficult decisions around engagement with employment are associated with parental well-being and functioning, if parenting a child in pain. If we cast parenting as occupation, then its job description is significantly changed by parenting a child in chronic pain, as this takes more effort, needs additions to the parenting skillset, and is associated with poorer parental well-being outcomes. However, we need to know much more about how to support parents in their own specific familial and work contexts, whatever those may be.

Turning to young people, Calnan and Douglass in Chapter 2 discuss how those in the youth labour market appear to be moving in to a more uncertain working environment, even before we consider the added impact of being a young person living with ongoing pain. Some human capital theories suggest that the more educated a young person is, the more productive and well remunerated they will be (Brown et al., 2011). More young people are well qualified than ever before yet a recent UK Office of National Statistics report shows that underemployment amongst graduates rose sharply between 2001 and 2013 (ONS, 2017). Calnan and Douglass suggest this trend can be explained by the marketization and deregulation accompanying globalization, such that there may be a mismatch between expectations and employment, and an international auction for highly skilled jobs. This situation is challenging for anyone to negotiate, let alone a young person also having to manage fluctuating levels of pain and functioning.

Fisher and Eccleston in Chapter 6 show that we do not yet have a good understanding of how being a millennial in pain may affect one's work and life goals. We know little about how millennials in pain receive, give, or co-produce health care. It is difficult, therefore, to apply the evidence base that 'good' work, or occupation more broadly, is good for most of us, including people in pain, directly to millennials. It is likely that 'good' work is good for millennials in pain in the same ways as it is for other generations. However, we need to rise to the opportunity to understand the broader sociological and psychological impact of being a millennial in pain and how this may affect the expectation of what good work is, including that millennials will likely have longer working lives and may prefer portfolio careers. For example, Fisher and Eccleston discuss how millennials may be better at challenging authority than other generations— does this extend to if they want a diagnosis for an ongoing pain condition, for example, or do not agree with the one they have got? Interestingly, Sullivan et al. in Chapter 9 argue that perceived injustice may be key to not doing well when trying to return to, or stay at, work with pain. We need to know more about this, such as how it may be linked in the transition from acute to chronic pain, and whether this could be linked to millennial willingness to challenge authority if there is a perceived injustice.

In Chapter 8, Eccleston presents a radical rethinking of later life production when one has pain, arguing that we must focus on understanding more about what kinds of occupation, assimilative goal pursuit, and accommodative adaption, might bolster positive identity management as we age. It may be possible to continue with, or return to, a previous occupation, but this may not be desirable or manageable for some people. So we need to comprehensively assess how new roles might be experimented with, and how occupational therapy could focus on valued and personally relevant roles, which could be in the context of extending one's working life, or concern more relational work such as caring.

Conceptualizing pain

Wainwright (Chapter 3) suggests that taking the embodied view of pain as action against uncertainty (see Eccleston 2016; Eccleston 2018; Tabor et al., 2017) means that if we are to reduce pain intrusion and interference, we must attend more deeply to how people manage threats to identity and coherence. We must consider how people manage this whilst they are at work, but also more broadly, since identity at work may well overlap with non-work identity. There is an opportunity to be appropriately creative about the ways in which we study how people (including young people) manage threats to identity. We could think about the role of cognitive intrusion and pain dominance in this respect, for example see work by Attridge et al. (2015). It may be helpful to think about the underlying mechanisms for identity management in relation to some of the key psychological variables implicated in return to work, as highlighted in Chapter 9 by Sullivan and colleagues. They discuss in compelling detail the need to know more about the cognitive risk factors (recovery expectancy, self-efficacy, catastrophizing, perceived injustice, and health beliefs) and mental health risk factors (depression and PTSD) in relation to work disability following musculoskeletal injury. For example, they discuss how outcome expectancies might represent the final common pathway of a variety of psychological influences on behaviour: we need to know more about how negative expectancies develop. It is possible that sufferers' verbalizations of negative expectancies might adversely impact the patient–healthcare practitioner alliance or that professionals are inadvertently helping to develop negative expectancies. It may be that low motivation linked to negative expectancies for pain sufferers leads to lack of participation in rehabilitation. We need to know more about the role of negative expectancies in how a pain sufferer experiences work, or more broadly, occupation, and whether this relates to how they manage identity and coherence. Furthermore, it would be useful to learn how a person's health beliefs and self-efficacy, also discussed as key by Sullivan et al., map on to efforts to managing threats to our identity and coherence when we live with pain.

Another useful way of conceptualizing pain at work is to consider whether the pain is occupational or not. This does not need to preclude the embodied view of pain as an action against uncertainty since whether or not the pain is occupational, people will probably be managing threats to identity and coherence (although if they know the pain is occupational this may change the quality of the perception of the threat). In Chapter 7, Verbeek makes a strong case for putting more resource into determining the (sometimes difficult) question of whether or not the pain is occupational, and suggests criteria by which this can be done. The distinction is important because if the pain is occupational, then instead of focusing on pain relief through medication and rest, workplace improvements can be proposed. Verbeek notes that the evidence for the relationship between adverse ergonomic factors and pain should come from a good systematic review from cohort studies that takes into account the factors that can confound the relationship but that these studies are few, so our roadmap here includes the recommendation for more such research. When a clear diagnosis of occupational pain has been ascertained, it would be useful to have high quality evidence that there are specific ergonomic improvements which can reduce the occupational pain in context. For example, Verbeek's dental technician needed better designed dental appliances. Even though there are many studies that propose ergonomic improvements, there are very few studies that have evaluated the effects of interventions on pain, so we need to know more about the effects of such ergonomic improvements. Linked to this, as Eccleston notes in Chapter 8 when thinking about later life production, sometimes a person will not have had an occupational and environmental assessment to see what could be changed around them. It is really important to consider this kind of support for someone in pain: whether this is at school and they are carrying heavy rucksacks full of textbooks, or they are working-aged as per Verbeek's dental technician, or they are a much older person; all could be helped to consider if there are ergonomic or environmental ways to improve occupational pain.

Future directions for research

Table 12.1 provides a summary of key domains and questions for taking a life-span approach to occupation and pain.

A focus on bi-directional relationships between parent and child with chronic pain

As Jordan and Jaaniste discuss, negative life experiences can be a significant predictor of change in a child's attachment relationship between infancy and adolescence (Hamilton, 2000). Whilst paediatric chronic pain is a stressor with a strong psychosocial component, so likely to lead to significant changes in parent–child relationships, we need more research in this area, especially as early parent–child relationships may form a template for future relationships (Malekpour, 2007). For example, can we support parents in parenting interventions which account for those specific personality factors and traits which when parenting a child with chronic pain, have been shown to be important (e.g. trait anxiety, pain-related catastrophizing, trait mindfulness, perfectionism, and empathy)? Although it may be hard to modify these factors, awareness of them may help parents, and also help clinicians trying to understand different parental responses. We highlight Jordan and Jaaniste's recommendation that future research should investigate the value of tailoring parent-based pain interventions to key parental personality factors.

Caes and Logan discussed that parental responses to pain can influence school functioning for young people with chronic pain, with parental negative thinking about pain having a mechanistic role (Logan, et al., 2012). We need to know more about how to support parents in this specific context of their child's schooling. However, Caes and Logan point out that school responses to child pain are also critical and we need further investigation into interactions between school responses to child pain, child functioning, and parental thinking about pain and about school.

The importance of a biopsychosocial approach to school functioning in young people and of elucidating key targets for intervention

Caes and Logan's proposed biopsychosocial model of school functioning in young people with chronic pain will enable us to research how pain, school functioning, and modulators of the pain–school functioning pathway, on both individual and systems levels, interact to shape the school experience in the context of chronic pain. The model should be applied and tested via different methods, including N of 1, cross-sectional, and longitudinal, and we should encourage further research with very young

Table 12.1 Next steps for research

Domains	Questions
Embodied pain	◆ How do people manage threats to identity and coherence when they are in pain in the context of work and occupation? ◆ How do attempts to manage pain interact with key psychological variables known to affect pain-related work disability?
Pain-related work limitations	◆ What are the behavioural determinants of the limitations of work? ◆ How open to change are these determinants? ◆ How can we redesign organizational, social, and personal interventions to promote behaviour change?
Treatment and prevention	◆ Can we define treatment as an intervention that is delivered at the request of the patient and prevention as something offered by the provider? ◆ Will this reduce cross-over between what might be considered treatment and what might be considered intervention?
Ergonomic intervention	◆ Can we use randomized controlled studies with patients complaining of occupational pain to discover whether ergonomic interventions have an effect on occupational pain? ◆ How do we facilitate larger studies to better understand the effects of prevention so we may then show any effects that can be used in prevention?
Consensus building	◆ How do we establish consensus about which disability and work participation outcomes we measure, and how to measure them, in work and pain studies? ◆ How might this consensus lead to better comparison between studies, developing the evidence base and informing policy making?
Intergenerational transfer	◆ What are the optimum parent-focused interventions for parental and child well-being when parenting a child in pain? ◆ Can we tailor interventions to key parental individual differences and parenting styles known to influence child–parent relationships when a child has pain? ◆ How can we tailor effective interventions to be developmentally appropriate to children? ◆ How can we help parents who are parenting a child in pain to engage with the labour market in order to maximize their own, and their child's, health outcomes? ◆ How can we help parents who are parenting a child in pain, and who also suffer themselves from pain, to negotiate these two pathways successfully and simultaneously? ◆ Is there a backward transmission of pain from a younger to an older person? ◆ How can we use research in this area to narrow gaps between generations about analgesic and pain beliefs and expectations? ◆ How can we promote intergenerational communication enabling positive beliefs about better coping and living a good life with chronic pain?

(continued)

Table 12.1   Continued

Domains	Questions
Development and education	◆ How can individual parents, class teachers, and schools at an organizational level best respond to a child in pain? ◆ How can such responses be tailored to children at all levels of education systems including pre-schoolers? ◆ How can end-of-school and earlier vocational, enterprise, and careers advice be tailored for young people in pain, at the same time as accounting for the specifics of modern labour markets? ◆ Can we recover developmental impairments associated with chronic pain, such as feeling socially delayed, both in and out of school settings?
Cognitive performance	◆ What is the impact of pain medication on cognitive functioning in children of different ages? ◆ What is the impact of analgesic medication on cognitive functioning as young people progress through different stages of occupation (e.g. university or other work as youths) and as they move towards middle age and later life production?
Later life production	◆ What meanings are assigned in later life to goals still pursued or put aside, including goals thought of traditionally as occupational? ◆ How we can make modern cognitive behavioural therapy approaches for people in later life living with chronic pain more socially and contextually relevant? ◆ How can not only psychological but also vocational and physiotherapy support be used to enable meaningful occupation? ◆ How do we make use of modern computing technology to increase access to therapy and to develop novel therapy?

and post-adolescent youth, since most research focuses on adolescents at present. Via testing and revision, the model should also enable elucidation of defined targets of intervention (as Caes and Logan note, for one young person the key to school success might be treating anxiety focused on the school setting, whereas for another it may be most important to help the teachers understand the pain issues and respond to the young person supportively). Conceptually, it is interesting to note links here between Caes and Logan's focus on the need for precision in intervention targets for children with that championed by Sullivan et al. in adults. They argue that we should invest more in finding out which psychological variables in adults contribute unique variance to predicting recovery from pain-related injury and hence which variables might interventions be specially designed to modify.

A life-course approach to reducing developmental impairments associated with chronic pain

Fisher and Eccleston discuss how we know that adolescents living with pain perceived themselves as socially delayed compared to their peers (Eccleston et al., 2008); higher pain-related anxiety specifically in female youth has been associated with impairment in the development of self-perception (Caes et al., 2015). We do not know if these perceptions of development can recover if pain is managed appropriately, and if treatment could be targeted for not only school age youth but also pre-schoolers and millennials, to help them manage some of the difficult psychological impacts of living with chronic pain.

Taking a lifespan approach towards academic performance in young people with pain, and later work performance

This approach is missing from the literature. It would allow us to answer key questions such as: What is the impact of repeated pain experiences in pre-schoolers on school performance, with a focus on when such impact first appears? As Caes and Logan discuss, there is evidence regarding how repeated pain experiences in neonates impacts their pain sensitivity later in childhood, but we urgently need longitudinal work to assess the impact of early pain exposure on neurodevelopment, and associated issues such as cognitive and academic outcomes. We also need longitudinal studies on the effects of impaired school performance (or early experience) on later academic or work performance. We know, for example, that factors such as self-efficacy, school attendance, and social and academic engagement, can predict long-term academic and career outcomes, but we know little about the potential negative effect of pain experiences on school functioning longitudinally, and how pain-related school impairments influence future academic, career and work opportunities and performance.

Caes and Logan's biopsychosocial model of school functioning in young people, and its attendant use to elucidate defined targets of intervention, relates to the discussion by Sullivan et al. regarding how we should invest more to discover which psychological variables in adults contribute unique variance to predicting recovery from pain-related injury and hence which might interventions be specially designed to modify. It appears that it would be very fruitful to investigate which psychological modulators of the pain-school and pain-work functioning pathways shape school and work experiences in the context of chronic pain. This should involve taking a life-span perspective so we can learn more about the determinants, determinant changers, and the modification of such variables over time. This also enables a focus on the later effects of very early years' pain experience, which is under-researched and yet critical to understand.

Taking a lifespan approach to role of analgesia when investigating cognitive functioning during occupation

Caes and Logan note that whilst there is some evidence that pain medication can contribute to poorer cognitive functioning (Moriarty et al., 2011), little research exists examining the impact of pain medication on cognitive functioning in paediatric populations. They point out the importance, therefore, of controlling for the effect of analgesics when investigating associations between paediatric chronic pain and school functioning. Similarly, we know little about the impact of analgesic medication on cognitive functioning in the context of being at work, for working age adults (and indeed for young people globally who may be doing different kinds of paid work very different to schooling, and from very young ages in some countries).

Wainwright noted in Chapter 3 that there is a body of research beginning to unpick how pain interferes with different kinds of cognition. Attridge et al. (2017) found that headache slows people down relative to when they are headache-free in multiple attention tasks, mostly those involving attentional switching or selective attention. This is important when we think about how pain impacts on work, and further, we need to know much more about the impact of the kinds of analgesic medication people might take to relieve headache (for example) on cognitive functioning whilst working. In addition, we need further investigation of the underlying mechanisms by which pain medication affects cognitive functioning for young people and workers, and we need to control for the effect of analgesics when investigating associations between paediatric pain and school functioning, and between adults of working age and their job functioning.

Applying knowledge to non-traditional patterns of work and occupation

We outlined above a summary of what 'good' work is for people in pain according to the expert contributors to this book. We also need to consider how we might apply all these parameters to those who are self-employed, for those working within the new precariat, and for older workers, all groups which are growing. For example, are the effects of pain worse or different for those in the precariat and conversely, is it harder to sustain a precariat working life when one lives with pain? Calnan and Douglass (Chapter 2) review how a combination of precarity, poor rights, and lack of access to appropriate occupational health provision means that so-called gig workers are often vulnerable to a higher risk of ill-health, particularly mental ill-health. For example, Pilgrim (2014) discussed research looking at the relationship between work and mental health that suggests that the worst mental health scores are not found in the unemployed but in those in insecure employment. Alternatively, could the precariat system actually enable pain sufferers to work in a way that suits them, (e.g. if they do not need to work full time for financial reasons, or if their skills are so highly valued in the market that they can get a high hourly rate) reaping the psychosocial and financial benefits of work without having to commit to a more traditional working role? The precariat are perhaps best henceforth referred to as the contingent workforce, since as Bevan notes in Chapter 11, not all may be precariously employed; being a courier is likely a very different experience in terms of power and money than being a specialist IT contractor. This creates distinct heterogeneity within this group. Similarly, there are many related questions we could ask about the self-employed, since very little attention has been paid to them in the literature on work and pain. Notably, Main and Shaw in Chapter 10 point out that the UK Fit for Work Service explicitly excluded them.

The intervention toolbox model (Kendall et al., 2015) has been built on the best available theory and evidence with regard to work-relevant common health problems and could be comprehensively tested with regard to sustaining working lives for people in pain. We also need to test how it may relate to the self-employed (who may not have line managers but still need a safe working environment and ability to modify job roles); to the contingent workforce with all their differing power and financial relations to employment; to millennials, who as discussed by Fisher and Eccleston in

Chapter 6 may have particular ways of responding to and creating occupation, and to those engaged in later life production, who may have different wants and needs from their younger counterparts. For example, Fisher and Eccleston argue that we cannot afford to miss gaining a better understanding of the broader sociological and psychological impact of being a millennial in pain. We need to work out how to apply this new knowledge to better equip line managers (who may be managing millennials, and more of whom will gradually be millennials themselves) with the tools to help millennials in pain in the workforce.

Calnan and Douglass in Chapter 2 and Wainwright in Chapter 3 discuss how the kinds of occupation in which we are engaged, our working conditions, and whether we want to work, may all affect how pain impacts on our working lives, and how our work may relate to the pain experience. We simply do not know enough about some relationships between pain and work, such as the effect on pain of working in a job we do not enjoy versus one we do, or of working primarily because of financial need versus for personal or social validation. Furthermore, we should consider these issues for the different kinds of worker populations elucidated above.

Future directions for policy

Table 12.2 provides a summary of policy areas and questions that we judge important in making the policy landscape better for people living with ongoing pain.

Table 12.2 Next steps for policy

Early intervention	◆ Can we develop and resource a new generation of nationally sponsored early intervention tools to support workers with pain and pain-related conditions to remain in work? ◆ For example, can we support screening for work instability, in which we may determine which aspects of someone's job elevate their risk of taking absence from work or even leaving work?
Compensation	◆ Can workers with disabilities from presumed or confirmed non-occupationally related pain access worker compensation schemes in different countries? ◆ How should financial considerations and duty of care be weighted within this decision?
Health technology appraisal	◆ Can work participation and productivity benefits be included in health technology appraisal to judge whether labour market participation improves?
Longitudinal approaches	◆ How can our political and policy-making systems be changed to enable policy-makers to take the long view? ◆ Can we encourage initiatives between Government departments that may not deliver within one electoral cycle? ◆ Alternatively, should we focus on longer-term collaborations between local agencies and Government with a view to highlighting the benefits of such relationships to policy-makers?

A symbiotic relationship between research and policy

There needs to be a deeper, more symbiotic relationship between research and policy. We accept this is challenging, but there is too much at stake not to rise to this challenge. Researchers are getting very good at showing policy-makers where the best evidence lies, particularly for large cohort studies, trials, and so on, although there are still relationships and systems to be built on both sides to encourage policy-makers to respond more quickly to progressing science. Researchers could do more to make policy-makers see the value of qualitative research, especially in areas where there is grey literature and where the research question at stake is best answered using a qualitative approach. We note the growing recognition of the importance and utility of qualitative work shown by policy-makers in different arenas, especially around issues such as the acceptance and feasibility of proposed interventions and policies by stakeholders: this is to be welcomed and could be further foregrounded in policy-making on pain and work.

Policy-makers need to be more responsive to changing scientific findings and be held to account if not using the best available evidence to answer the policy question. Researchers need to continue to work hard to engage policy-makers with high quality work. On the other hand, policy-makers also have an important part to play in expecting researchers to use common outcome measures, where appropriate, to enable better comparison of studies which can then inform policy. Verbeek makes a strong argument for gaining consensus about which disability and work participation outcomes should be measured and how to measure them. Policy-makers could expect these to be agreed measure to be used, where appropriate, in any work which is contributing to policy-making decisions.

Stronger use of evidence to inform policy

The chapters by Verbeek and Bevan both discuss difficulties with getting science into policy-thinking and policy-making. Bevan elucidates very good reasons why this is challenging, and Verbeek discusses that, for example, there is not very good evidence that a straight back is important in preventing back pain but that it has proven very difficult to remove this from policy even as the science has moved on. Verbeek argues that current regulation mandating certain workplace requirements should be informed by the best available evidence. We need to work to ensure that any preventative measures which are laid down in regulation are actually open to change as the science changes. For future policies and regulation, the regulatory body should include scientific evidence to underpin the effectiveness of the interventions mandated by the regulation. Ideally, this should be so even if things are presented as guidance rather than legislation. Regulation should be able to keep pace with advancing science around workplace changes and progressing knowledge of specific risks.

The need for longitudinal research: a policy issue too

Much research (especially into parenting a child with pain, and the effects of pain on schooling) is cross-sectional, yet we urgently need longitudinal research so, for example, we can assess the impacts of the qualitative changes in the developing child in pain on the child–parent dyad, or the effects of impaired school performance, or early experience, on later academic or work experience. As Chapters 4 and 5 point out, we have very little longitudinal data on these two topics and yet, how important it is that we do explore them, so that we can then start to design ways to reduce barriers for children in pain to achieving ongoing secure attachment, and positive academic and work outcomes. We know that longitudinal research is imperfect (e.g. key questions within a topic may change over time), but it is still useful in many situations (e.g. to enable better knowledge about how millennials search for and use health care information, as they become a dominant force in society). However, longitudinal research requires the money and political will to get beyond election terms, and consider a much longer-term cost–benefit framework (as Bevan discusses). Bevan considers that the challenges in adopting such a perspective are so great within current systems that it may be more realistic to consider alternatives such as budget pooling. Although we agree with Bevan about the scale of the challenge before us, and admire the promising results for budget pooling, we invite policy-makers to consider the value of longitudinal research projects about interactions between occupation and pain; the potential gains are great.

Workplace policies: regulation or latitude?

Two key inter-linked themes arise from this book. First, Main and Shaw (Chapter 10) note that since workplace policies typically find it hard to accommodate the intermittent pattern of work absence that can occur with chronic pain, an employee-driven approach may enable a more responsive paradigm rather than having to make formal requests for accommodation each time function shifts. However, Bevan discusses how different policy-making systems allow for more or less regulation in particular areas. He gives the particular example of how employers respond to the contingent workforce about job role modification. We need to systematically compare different degrees of regulation versus latitude regarding exactly how employers are able to respond to job role modification. For example, what would happen if an employee-driven approach was mandated? How would this work for different kinds of organizations? How would this work for the contingent workforce? Conversely, what would be the benefits and drawbacks of allowing latitude with regard to how an organization responds to fluctuating function but putting in place incentives (not necessarily financial) to enable an employee-driven system?

More broadly, Bevan (Chapter 10) relates the evidence that good work is good for us, to a more regulatory framework in the UK, which is now moving beyond health and safety towards enforcement of a better consideration of worker well-being. Might it be mandated that employers need to fulfil legal (and moral) duties of care towards employers, so the direction of travel is clear, but the precise execution within organizations is left very open, via the flexible, employee-centred approach suggested by Main and Shaw?

Conclusion

We have shown the importance of taking a life-span approach to reducing impairment associated with chronic pain, to academic performance in young people with pain, and later work performance, and to the role of analgesia in cognitive function. We have also argued for the importance of taking a life-span approach when studying interactions between pain and occupation, since we need to know more about how these are shaped by being very young, by being a millennial, and by being at work post-retirement age, in addition to being an adolescent and being an adult of working, non-pensionable age, which are the two groups most often studied. Included in such an approach can be very different forms of occupation, such as schooling, parenting, contingent working, self-employment, and later life production. All these need further studying so that we can enable everyone who wants or needs to participate in the labour market and in other forms of occupation to do so to the best of their ability, in systems which can encompass fluctuations in pain. The need to help people in pain will not weaken, but rather is set to increase as we become more knowledgeable at one end of the spectrum about the lasting effects of pain in childhood, and at the other, are more prescient of the demands of an aging population. From childhood and adolescence to millennials and beyond **it is important that we take a life-course approach to occupation and work when in pain**. Through a better understanding of how and why people seek to be occupied, we can help people maximize their social and personal involvement. We hope you will join us in our call to improve knowledge about interactions between pain and occupation, so we can act to reduce the multifaceted suffering caused by living with ongoing pain.

References

Attridge, N., Crombez, G., Van Ryckeghem, D., Keogh, E., and Eccleston, C. (2015) The Experience of Cognitive Intrusion of Pain: scale development and validation. *Pain*, **156**, 1978.

Attridge, N., Eccleston, C., Noonan, D., Wainwright, E., and Keogh, E. (2017) Headache impairs attentional performance: a conceptual replication and extension. *The Journal of Pain*, **18**, 29–41.

Brown, P., Lauder, H., and Ashton, D. (2011) *The Global Auction: The Broken Promises of Education, Jobs and Incomes*. Oxford: Oxford University Press

Caes, L., Fisher, E., Clinch, J., Tobias, J. H., and Eccleston, C. (2015) The role of pain related anxiety in adolescents' disability and social impairment: ALSPAC data. *European Journal of Pain*, **19**, 842–51.

Eccleston, C. (2016) *Embodied: the Psychology of Physical Sensation*. Oxford: Oxford University Press.

Eccleston, C. (2018) Chronic pain as embodied defence: implications for current and future psychological treatments. *Pain*, **159**, Suppl 1, S17–23.

Eccleston, C., Wastell, S., Crombez, G., and Jordan, A. 2008. Adolescent social development and chronic pain. *European Journal of Pain*, **12**, 765–74

Hamilton, C. E. (2000) Continuity and discontinuity of attachment from infancy through adolescence. *Child Development*, **71**, 690–4.

Kendall, N., Burton, A. K., Lunt, J., Mellor, N., and Daniels, K. (2015) *The HSE Toolbox Developing an Intervention Toolbox for Common Health Problems in the Workplace*. London: HSE Books.

Logan, D. E., Simons, L. E., and **Carpino, E. A.** (2012) Too sick for school? Parent influences on school functioning among children with chronic pain. *Pain*, **153**, 437–43.

Logan, D. E., and **Curran, J. A.** (2005) Adolescent chronic pain problems in the school setting: Exploring the experiences and beliefs of selected school personnel through focus group methodology. *Journal of Adolescent Health*, 37, 281–8.

Malekpour, M. (2007) Effects of attachment on early and later development. *British Journal of Development Disabilities*, **53**, 81–95.

Mann, A., and **Huddleston, P.** (2017) Schools and the twenty-first century labour market: Perspectives on structural change. *British Journal of Guidance and Counselling*, **45,** 208–18.

Moriarty, O., McGuire, B. E., and **Finn, D. P.** (2011) The effect of pain on cognitive function: a review of clinical and preclinical research. *Progress in Neurobiology*, **93**, 385–404.

Office of National Statistics (2017) Graduates in the Labour Market Office, November. Online. Available at: https://www.ons.gov.uk/releases/graduatesintheuklabourmarket2017 [Accessed 22nd March 2019]

Palermo, T. M., Law, E. F., Bromberg, M., Fales, J., Eccleston, C., and **Wilson, A. C.** (2016) Problem-solving skills training for parents of children with chronic pain. *Pain*, **157**, 1213–23.

Pilgrim, D. (2014) *Key Concepts in Mental Health.* Third Edition. Thousand Oaks: Sage.

Shaw W.S., van der Windt, D. A. W., Main, C. J., Loisel, P., and **Linton, S. J.** (2009) Now tell me about your work: the feasibility of early screening and intervention to address occupational factors ("Blue Flags") in back disability. *Journal of Occupational Rehabilitation*, **19**, 64–80.

Tabor, A., Keogh, E., and **Eccleston, C.** (2017) Embodied pain—negotiating the boundaries of possible action. *Pain*, **158**, 1007–11.

Tarpey, S. L., Caes, L., and **Heary, C.** (2018) Supporting children with chronic pain in school: Understanding teachers' experiences of pain in the classroom. *European Health Psychologist*, **20**, 419–24.

Waddell, G., and **Burton, A. K.** (2006) Is work good for your health and well-being? London: The Stationery Office.

Index

Note: Tables, figures, and boxes are indicated by *t*, *f*, and *b* following the page number
For the benefit of digital users, indexed terms that span two pages (e.g., 52–53) may, on occasion, appear on only one of those pages.